P9-DNA-651

Lippincott's Photo Atlas of Medication Administration

Lippincott's Photo Atlas of Medication Administration

Pamela Lynn, RN, MSN
Faculty
School of Nursing
Gwynedd-Mercy College
Gwynedd Valley, Pennsylvania

 Wolters Kluwer | Lippincott Williams & Wilkins
Health

Philadelphia • Baltimore • New York • London
Buenos Aires • Hong Kong • Sydney • Tokyo

Copyright © 2008 by Lippincott Williams & Wilkins, a Wolters Kluwer business.

All rights reserved. This book is protected by copyright. No part of it may be reproduced, stored in a retrieval system, or transmitted, in any form or by any means—electronic, mechanical, photocopy, recording, or otherwise—without prior written permission of the publisher, except for brief quotations embodied in critical articles and reviews and testing and evaluation materials provided by publisher to instructors whose schools have adopted its accompanying textbook. Printed in the United States of America. For information write Lippincott Williams & Wilkins, 530 Walnut Street, Philadelphia PA 19106.

Materials appearing in this book prepared by individuals as part of their official duties as U.S. Government employees are not covered by the above-mentioned copyright.

9 8 7 6 5 4 3 2 1

ISBN-13: 978-0-7817-6923-5
ISBN-10: 0-7817-6923-X

Care has been taken to confirm the accuracy of the information presented and to describe generally accepted practices. However, the author, editors, and publisher are not responsible for errors or omissions or for any consequences from application of the information in this book and make no warranty, express or implied, with respect to the content of the publication.

The author, editors, and publisher have exerted every effort to ensure that drug selection and dosage set forth in this text are in accordance with the current recommendations and practice at the time of publication. However, in view of ongoing research, changes in government regulations, and the constant flow of information relating to drug therapy and drug reactions, the reader is urged to check the package insert for each drug for any change in indications and dosage and for added warnings and precautions. This is particularly important when the recommended agent is a new or infrequently employed drug.

Some drugs and medical devices presented in this publication have Food and Drug Administration (FDA) clearance for limited use in restricted research settings. It is the responsibility of the health care provider to ascertain the FDA status of each drug or device planned for use in his or her clinical practice.

LWW.com

Contents

Administering Oral Medications

Drugs given orally are intended for absorption in the stomach and small intestine. The oral route is the most commonly used route of administration. It is usually the most convenient and comfortable for the patient. After oral administration, drug action has a slower onset and a more prolonged but less potent effect than other routes.

Equipment

- Medication in disposable cup or oral syringe
- Liquid (water, juice, etc.) with straw if not contraindicated
- Medication cart or tray
- Medication Administration Record (MAR) or Computer-generated MAR (CMAR)

ASSESSMENT

Assess the appropriateness of the drug for the patient. Review medical history, allergy, assessment, and laboratory data that may influence drug administration. Assess the patient's ability to swallow medications. If the patient cannot swallow, is NPO, or is experiencing nausea or vomiting, the medication should be withheld, the physician notified, and proper documentation completed. Assess the patient's knowledge of the medication. If the patient has a knowledge deficit about the medication, this may be the appropriate time to begin education about the medication. If the medication may affect the patient's vital signs, assess them before administration. If the medication is for pain relief, assess the patient's pain level before and after administration. Verify the patient name, dose, route, and time of administration.

NURSING DIAGNOSIS

Determine related factors for the nursing diagnoses based on the patient's current status. Appropriate nursing diagnoses may include:

- Impaired Swallowing
- Risk for Aspiration
- Anxiety
- Deficient Knowledge
- Noncompliance

OUTCOME IDENTIFICATION AND PLANNING

The expected outcome to achieve when administering an oral medication is that the patient will swallow the medication. Other outcomes that may be appropriate include the following: the patient will experience the desired effect from the medication; the patient will not aspirate; the patient experiences decreased anxiety; the patient does not experience adverse effects; and the patient understands and complies with the medication regimen.

IMPLEMENTATION

ACTION

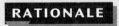
RATIONALE

1. Gather equipment. Check each medication order against the original physician's order according to agency policy. Clarify any inconsistencies. Check the patient's chart for allergies.

2. Know the actions, special nursing considerations, safe dose ranges, purpose of administration, and adverse effects of the medications to be administered. Consider the appropriateness of the medication for this patient.

This comparison helps to identify errors that may have occurred when orders were transcribed. The physician's order is the legal record of medication orders for each agency.

This knowledge aids the nurse in evaluating the therapeutic effect of the medication in relation to the patient's disorder and can also be used to educate the patient about the medication.

(continued)

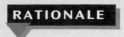

ACTION	RATIONALE

 3. Perform hand hygiene.

Hand hygiene prevents the spread of microorganisms.

4. Move the medication cart to the outside of the patient's room or prepare for administration in the medication area.

Organization facilitates error-free administration and saves time.

5. Unlock the medication cart or drawer. Enter pass code and scan employee identification, if required.

Locking of the cart or drawer safeguards each patient's medication supply. Hospital accrediting organizations require medication carts to be locked when not in use. Entering pass code and scanning ID allows only authorized users into the system and identifies user for documentation by the computer.

6. **Prepare medications for one patient at a time.**

This prevents errors in medication administration.

7. Read the MAR and select the proper medication from the patient's medication drawer or unit stock.

This is the first check of the label.

8. Compare the label with the MAR (Figure 1). Check expiration dates and perform calculations, if necessary. Scan the bar code on the package, if required.

This is the second check of the label. Verify calculations with another nurse to ensure safety, if necessary.

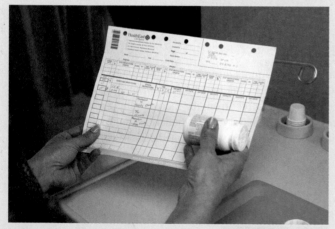

Figure 1. Comparing medication label with the MAR.

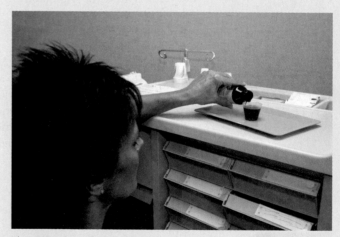

Figure 2. Measuring at eye level.

9. **Prepare the required medications:**

a. *Unit dose packages:* Place unit dose-packaged medications in a disposable cup. **Do not open wrapper until at the bedside.** Keep narcotics and medications that require special nursing assessments in a separate container.

Wrapper is kept intact because the label is needed for an additional safety check. Special assessments may be required before giving certain medications. These may include assessing vital signs and checking laboratory test results.

b. *Multidose containers:* When removing tablets or capsules from a multidose bottle, pour the necessary number into the bottle cap and then place the tablets in a medication cup. Break only scored tablets, if necessary, to obtain the proper dosage. Do not touch tablets with hands.

Pouring medication into the cap allows for easy return of excess medication to bottle. Pouring tablets or capsules into the nurse's hand is unsanitary.

Administering Oral Medications *(continued)*

ACTION

c. *Liquid medication in multidose bottle:* When pouring liquid medications in a multidose bottle, hold the bottle so the label is against the palm. Use the appropriate measuring device when pouring liquids, and read the amount of medication at the bottom of the meniscus at eye level (Figure 2). Wipe the lip of the bottle with a paper towel.

10. **When all medications for one patient have been prepared, recheck the label with the MAR before taking them to the patient. Replace any multidose containers in the patient's drawer or unit stock. Lock the medication cart before leaving it.**

11. Transport medications to the patient's bedside carefully, and keep the medications in sight at all times.

12. **Ensure that the patient receives the medications at the correct time.**

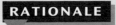

13. **Identify the patient.** Usually, the patient should be identified using two methods. Compare information with the MAR or CMAR.

a. Check the name and identification number on the patient's identification band (Figure 3).

b. Ask the patient to state his or her name.

c. If the patient cannot identify him or herself, verify the patient's identification with a staff member who knows the patient for the second source.

RATIONALE

Liquid that may drip onto the label makes the label difficult to read. Accuracy is possible when the appropriate measuring device is used and then read accurately.

This is a *third* check to ensure accuracy and to prevent errors. Locking the cart or drawer safeguards the patient's medication supply. Hospital accrediting organizations require medication carts to be locked when not in use.

Careful handling and close observation prevent accidental or deliberate disarrangement of medications.

Check agency policy, which may allow for administration within a period of 30 minutes before or 30 minutes after designated time.

Identifying the patient ensures the right patient receives the medications and helps prevent errors.

This is the most reliable method. Replace the identification band if it is missing or inaccurate in any way.

This requires a response from the patient, but illness and strange surroundings often cause patients to be confused.

This is another way to double check identity. Do not use the name on the door or over the bed, because these may be inaccurate.

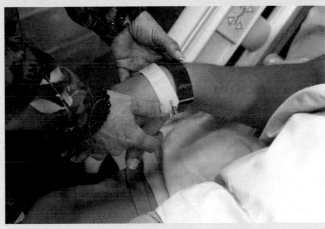

Figure 3. Checking patient's name and ID number.

(continued)

Administering Oral Medications (continued)

ACTION

RATIONALE

14. **Complete necessary assessments before administering medications. Check allergy bracelet or ask patient about allergies. Explain the purpose and action of each medication to the patient.**

Assessment is a prerequisite to administration of medications.

15. Scan the patient's bar code on the identification band, if required.

The bar code provides an additional check to ensure that the medication is given to the right patient.

16. Assist the patient to an upright or lateral position.

Swallowing is facilitated by proper positioning. An upright or side-lying position protects the patient from aspiration.

17. Administer medications:

  a. Offer water or other permitted fluids with pills, capsules, tablets, and some liquid medications.

Liquids facilitate swallowing of solid drugs. Some liquid drugs are intended to adhere to the pharyngeal area, in which case liquid is not offered with the medication.

  b. Ask whether the patient prefers to take the medications by hand or in a cup.

This encourages the patient's participation in taking the medications.

18. **Remain with the patient until each medication is swallowed. Never leave medication at the patient's bedside (Figure 4).**

Unless the nurse has seen the patient swallow the drug, the drug cannot be recorded as administered. The patient's chart is a legal record. Only with a physician's order can medications be left at the bedside.

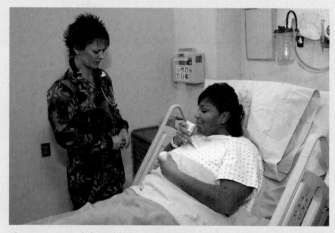

Figure 4. Remaining with the patient until each medication is swallowed.

19. Perform hand hygiene. Leave the patient in a comfortable position.

Hand hygiene prevents the spread of microorganisms.

20. Check on the patient within 30 minutes, or time appropriate for drug(s), to verify response to medication.

This provides the opportunity for further documentation and additional assessment of effectiveness of pain relief and adverse effects of medications.

Administering Oral Medications *(continued)*

EVALUATION

The expected outcomes are met when the patient swallows the medication, does not aspirate, verbalizes an understanding of the medication, experiences the desired effect from the medication, and does not experience adverse effects.

DOCUMENTATION

Guidelines

Record each medication given on the MAR or record using the required format immediately after it is administered, including date and time of administration (Figure 5). If using a bar-code system, medication administration is automatically recorded when scanned. PRN medications require documentation of the reason for administration. Prompt recording avoids the possibility of accidentally repeating the administration of the drug. If the drug was refused or omitted, record this in the appropriate area on the medication record and notify the physician. This verifies the reason medication was omitted and ensures that the physician is aware of the patient's condition. Recording of administration of a narcotic may require additional documentation on a narcotic record, stating drug count and other specific information. Record fluid intake if intake and output measurement is required.

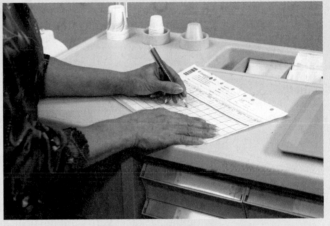

Figure 5. Recording each medication given on the MAR.

Sample Documentation

8/6/08 0835 Mr. Jones complaining of leg pains. Rates pain as an 8/10. Percocet 2 tabs administered.—K. Sanders, RN

8/6/08 0905 Mr. Jones resting comfortably. Rates leg pain as a 1/10.—K. Sanders, RN

8/6/08 1300 Mr. Jones refusing to take pain medication. States, "It made me feel woozy last time." Feelings discussed with patient. Patient agrees to take Percocet 1 tab at this time.—K. Sanders, RN

8/6/08 1320 Percocet, 1 tablet given P.O.—K. Sanders, RN

Unexpected Situations and Associated Interventions

- *Patient feels that medication is lodged in throat:* Offer patient more fluids to drink. If allowed, offer the patient bread or crackers to help move the medication to stomach.
- *It is unclear whether patient swallowed medication:* Check in the patient's mouth, under tongue, and between cheek and gum. Patients may "cheek" medications to avoid taking the medication or to save it for later use. This has been established with many medications, especially antidepressants and pain medication. Patients requiring suicide precautions should be watched closely to ensure that they are not "cheeking" the medication or hiding it in the mouth. These patients may be trying to accumulate a large amount of medication to take all at once in a suicide attempt. Substance abusers may cheek medication to accumulate a large amount to take all at once so that they may feel a high from medication.

(continued)

- *Patient vomits immediately or shortly after receiving oral medication:* Assess vomit, looking for pills or fragments. Do not readminister medication without notifying physician. If a whole pill is seen and can be identified, physician may ask that medication be administered again. If a pill is not seen or medications cannot be identified, medication should not be readministered so that patient does not receive too large a dose.
- *Child refuses to take oral medications:* Some medications may be mixed in a small amount of food, such as pudding or ice cream. Do not add to liquid, because medication may alter the taste of liquids; if child then refuses to drink the rest of the liquid, you will not know how much of the medication was ingested. Creativity may be needed when devising ways to administer medications to a child. See below under "Infant and Child Considerations" for suggestions.
- *The capsule or tablet falls to the floor during administration.* Discard and obtain a new dose for administration. This prevents contamination and transmission of microorganisms.
- *Patient refuses medication.* Explore the reason for the patient's refusal. Review the rationale for using the drug and any other information that may be appropriate. If you are unable to administer the medication despite education and discussion, document the omission according to facility policy and notify the physician.

Special Considerations

General Considerations

- Some liquid medication preparations, such as suspensions, require agitation to ensure even distribution of medication in the solution. Be familiar with the specific requirements for medications you are administering.
- Medications intended for sublingual absorption should be placed under the patient's tongue. Instruct the patient to allow the medication to dissolve completely. Reinforce the importance of not swallowing the medication tablet.
- Some oral medications are provided in powdered forms. Verify the correct liquid to dissolve the medication in for administration. This information is usually included on the package; verify any unclear instructions with a pharmacist or medication reference. If there is more than one possible liquid to dissolve the medication in, include the patient in the decision process; patients may find one choice more palatable than another.
- Ongoing assessment is an important part of nursing care to evaluate patient response to administered medications and early detection of adverse effects. If an adverse effect is suspected, withhold further medication doses and notify the patient's primary healthcare provider. Additional intervention is based on type of reaction and patient assessment.
- If the patient questions a medication order or states the medication is different from the usual dose, always recheck and clarify with the original order or physician before giving medication.
- If the patient's level of consciousness is altered or his or her swallowing is impaired, check with the physician to clarify the route of administration or alternative forms of medication. This may also be a solution for a pediatric or a confused patient who is refusing to take a medication.
- Patients with poor vision can request large-type labels on medication containers. A magnifying lens also may be helpful.
- Provide written medication information to reinforce discussion and education, if the patient is literate. If the patient is unable to read, provide written information to family or significant other, if appropriate. Written information should be at a 5th-grade level to ensure ease of understanding.

Administering Oral Medications *(continued)*

- If the patient has difficulty swallowing tablets, it may be appropriate to crush the medication to facilitate administration. Not all medications can be crushed or altered. Consult a medication reference and/or pharmacist. Long-acting and slow-release drugs are examples of medications that cannot be crushed. If the medication can be crushed, use a pill-crusher or mortar and pestle to grind the tablet into a powder. Crush each pill one at a time. Dissolve the powder with water or other recommended liquid in a liquid medication cup, keeping each medication separate from the others. Keep the package label with the medication cup for future comparison of information. The medication can then be combined with small amount of soft food, such as applesauce or pudding, to facilitate administration.

Infant and Child Considerations

- Special devices, such as oral syringes and calibrated nipples, are available in a pharmacy to ensure accurate dose calculations for young children and infants.
- Some creative ways to administer medications to children include: have a "tea party" with medicine cups; place syringe (without needle) or dropper in the space between the cheek and gum and slowly administer the medication; save a special treat for after the medication administration (eg, movie, playroom time, or a special food if allowed).
- The FDA has received reports of infants choking on the plastic caps that fit on the end of syringes when used to administer oral medications. They recommend the following: remove and dispose of caps before giving syringes to patients or families, caution family caregivers to dispose of caps on syringes they buy over the counter, and report any problems with syringe caps to the FDA. Companies have begun to manufacture syringes labeled "oral use" without the caps on them.

Older Adult Considerations

- Elderly patients with arthritis may have difficulty opening childproof caps. On request, the pharmacist can substitute a cap that is easier to open. A rubber band twisted around the cap may provide a more secure grip for older patients.
- Consider large-print written information when appropriate.

Home Care Considerations

- Encourage the patient to discard outdated prescription medications.
- Discuss safe storage of medications when there are children and pets in the environment.
- Discuss with parents the difference in over-the-counter medications made for infants and medications made for children. Many times parents do not realize that there are different strengths to the actual medications, leading to under- or overdosing.
- Encourage patients to carry a card listing all medications, dosage, and frequency in case of an emergency.
- Discuss the importance of using an appropriate measuring device for liquid medications. Patients should be cautioned not to use eating utensils for measuring medications. A liquid medication cup, oral syringe, or measuring spoon should be used to provide accurate dosing.

Removing Medication From an Ampule

An ampule is a glass flask that contains a single dose of medication for parenteral adminis-tration. Because there is no way to prevent airborne contamination of any unused portion of medication after the ampule is opened, if not all the medication is used, the remainder must be discarded. Medication is removed from an ampule after its thin neck is broken.

Equipment

- Sterile syringe and filter needle
- Ampule of medication
- Small gauze pad
- Medication Administration Record (MAR) or Computer-generated MAR (CMAR)

ASSESSMENT

Assess the medication in the ampule for any particles or discoloration. Assess the ampule for any cracks or chips. Check expiration date before administering the medication. Verify patient name, dose, route, and time of administration. Assess the appropriateness of the drug for the patient. Review assessment and laboratory data that may influence drug administration.

NURSING DIAGNOSIS

Determine related factors for the nursing diagnoses based on the patient's current status. Appropriate nursing diagnoses may include:

- Risk for Infection
- Risk for Injury
- Anxiety
- Deficient Knowledge

OUTCOME IDENTIFICATION AND PLANNING

The expected outcome to achieve when removing medication from an ampule is that the medication will be removed in a sterile manner, be free from glass shards, and the proper dose is prepared.

IMPLEMENTATION

ACTION

RATIONALE

1. Gather equipment. Check the medication order against the original physician's order according to agency pol-icy. Clarify any inconsistencies. Check the patient's chart for allergies.

   This comparison helps to identify errors that may have occurred when orders were transcribed. The physician's order is the legal record of medication orders for each agency.

2. Know the actions, special nursing considerations, safe dose ranges, purpose of administration, and adverse ef-fects of the medications to be administered. Consider the appropriateness of the medication for this patient.

   This knowledge aids the nurse in evaluating the therapeutic effect of the medication in relation to the patient's dis-order and can also be used to educate the patient about the medication.

 3. Perform hand hygiene.

   Hand hygiene deters the spread of microorganisms.

4. Move the medication cart to the outside of the patient's room or prepare for administration in the medication area.

   Organization facilitates error-free administration and saves time.

Removing Medication From an Ampule *(continued)*

ACTION

5. Unlock the medication cart or drawer. Enter pass code and scan employee identification, if required.

6. **Prepare medications for one patient at a time.**

7. Read the MAR and select the proper medication from the patient's medication drawer or unit stock.

8. Compare the label with the MAR. Check expiration dates and perform calculations, if necessary. Scan the bar code on the package, if required.

9. Tap the stem of the ampule (Figure 1) or twist your wrist quickly (Figure 2) while holding the ampule vertically.

10. **Wrap a small gauze pad around the neck of the ampule.**

11. Use a snapping motion to break off the top of the ampule along the scored line at its neck (Figure 3). Always break away from your body.

RATIONALE

Locking of the cart or drawer safeguards each patient's medication supply. Hospital accrediting organizations require medication carts to be locked when not in use. Entering pass code and scanning ID allows only authorized users into the system and identifies user for documentation by the computer.

This prevents errors in medication administration.

This is the first check of the label.

This is the second check of the label. Verify calculations with another nurse to ensure safety, if necessary.

This facilitates movement of medication in the stem to the body of the ampule.

This protects the nurse's fingers from the glass as the ampule is broken.

This protects the nurse's face and fingers from any shattered glass fragments.

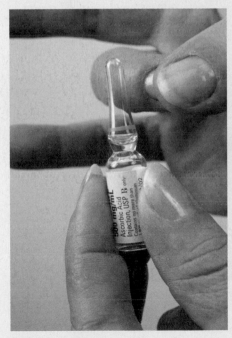
Figure 1. Tapping stem of the ampule.

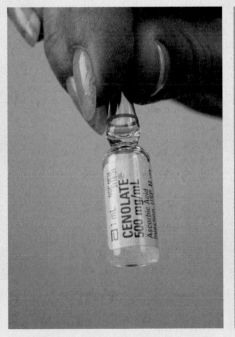
Figure 2. Twisting wrist quickly while holding the ampule vertically.

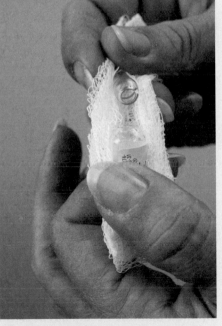
Figure 3. Using a snapping motion to break top of the ampule.

(continued)

ACTION

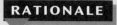

RATIONALE

12. Attach filter needle to syringe. **Remove the cap from the filter needle by pulling it straight off. Insert the filter needle into the ampule, being careful not to touch the rim.**

13. Withdraw medication in the amount ordered plus a small amount more (approximately 30%). **Do not inject air into the solution.** Use either of the following methods:

    a. Insert the tip of the needle into the ampule, which is upright on a flat surface, and withdraw fluid into the syringe (Figure 4). **Touch plunger at knob only.**

    b. Insert the tip of the needle into the ampule and invert the ampule (Figure 5). Keep the needle centered and not touching the sides of the ampule. Withdraw fluid into syringe. **Touch plunger at knob only.**

The rim of the ampule is considered contaminated. Use of a filter needle prevents the accidental withdrawing of small glass particles with the medication.

By withdrawing a small amount more of medication, any air bubbles in the syringe can be displaced once the syringe is removed and there will still be ample medication in the syringe.

The contents of the ampule are not under pressure; therefore, air is unnecessary and will cause the contents to overflow. Handling plunger at knob only will keep shaft of plunger sterile.

Surface tension holds the fluids in the ampule when inverted. If the needle touches the sides or is removed and then reinserted into the ampule, surface tension is broken, and fluid runs out. Handling plunger at knob only will keep shaft of plunger sterile.

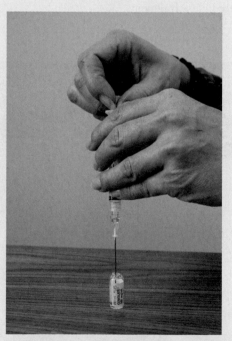

Figure 4. Withdrawing medication from upright ampule.

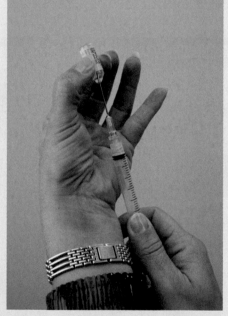

Figure 5. Withdrawing medication from inverted ampule.

14. **Wait until the needle has been withdrawn to tap the syringe and expel the air carefully by pushing on the plunger. Check the amount of medication in the syringe with the medication dose and discard any surplus according to facility policy.**

15. **Recheck the label with the MAR.**

Ejecting air into the solution increases pressure in the ampule and can force the medication to spill out over the ampule. Ampules may have overfill. Careful measurement ensures that correct dose is withdrawn.

This is the *third* check to ensure accuracy and to prevent errors.

Removing Medication From an Ampule *(continued)*

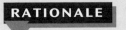

ACTION

16. Engage safety guard on filter needle and remove. Discard the filter needle in a suitable container. Attach appropriate administration device to syringe.

17. Discard the ampule in a suitable container.

18. Lock the medication cart before leaving it.

 19. Perform hand hygiene.

20. Proceed with administration, based on prescribed route.

RATIONALE

Filter needle used to draw up medication should not be used to administer the medication, to prevent any glass shards from entering the patient.

Any medication that has not been removed from the ampule must be discarded because there is no way to maintain sterility of contents in an opened ampule.

Locking the cart or drawer safeguards the patient's medication supply. Hospital accrediting organizations require medication carts to be locked when not in use.

Hand hygiene deters the spread of microorganisms.

See appropriate skill for prescribed route.

EVALUATION

The expected outcome is met when the medication is removed from the ampule in a sterile manner, free from glass shards, and the proper dose is prepared.

Unexpected Situations and Associated Interventions

- *Nurse cuts self while trying to open ampule:* Discard ampule in case contamination has occurred. Bandage wound and obtain a new ampule. Report according to agency policy.
- *All of medication was not removed from the stem and there is not enough medication left in body of ampule for dose:* Discard ampule and drawn medication. Obtain a new ampule and start over. Medication in original ampule stem is considered contaminated once neck of ampule has been placed on a nonsterile surface.
- *Nurse injects air into inverted ampule, spraying medication:* Wash hands to remove any medication. If any medication has gotten into eyes, perform eye irrigation. Obtain a new ampule for medication dose. Report injury, if necessary, according to agency policy.
- *Medication is drawn up without using a filter needle:* Replace needle with a filter needle. Inject the medication through the filter needle into a new syringe and then administer to patient.
- *Plunger becomes contaminated before inserted into ampule:* Discard needle and syringe and start over. If plunger is contaminated after medication is drawn into the syringe, it is not necessary to discard and start over. The contaminated plunger will enter the barrel of the syringe when pushing the medication out and will not contaminate the medication.

SKILL 3

Removing Medication From a Vial

A vial is a glass bottle with a self-sealing stopper through which medication is removed. For safety in transporting and storing, the vial top is usually covered with a soft metal cap that can be removed easily. The self sealing stopper that is then exposed is the means of entrance into the vial. Single-dose vials are used once, then discarded, regardless of the amount of the drug that is used from the vial. Multidose vials contain several doses of medication and can be used multiple times. The medication contained in a vial can be in liquid or powder form. Powdered forms must be dissolved in an appropriate diluent before administration. The following skill reviews removing liquid medication from a vial. Refer to the accompanying Skill Variation for steps to reconstitute a powdered medication.

Equipment

- Sterile syringe and needle or blunt cannula (size depends on medication being administered and patient)
- Vial of medication
- Antimicrobial swab
- Second needle (optional)
- Filter needle (optional)
- Medication Administration Record (MAR) or Computer-generated MAR (CMAR)

ASSESSMENT

Assess the medication in vial for any discoloration or particles. Check expiration date before administering medication. Assess the appropriateness of the drug for the patient. Review assessment and laboratory data that may influence drug administration. Verify the patient name, dose, route, and time of administration.

NURSING DIAGNOSIS

Determine related factors for the nursing diagnoses based on the patient's current status. Appropriate nursing diagnoses include:

- Risk for Infection.
- Risk for Injury
- Anxiety
- Deficient Knowledge

OUTCOME IDENTIFICATION AND PLANNING

The expected outcome to achieve when removing medication from a vial is withdrawal of the medication into a syringe in a sterile manner and that the proper dose is prepared.

IMPLEMENTATION

ACTION

1. Gather equipment. Check the medication order against the original physician's order according to agency policy.

2. Know the actions, special nursing considerations, safe dose ranges, purpose of administration, and adverse effects of the medications to be administered. Consider the appropriateness of the medication for this patient.

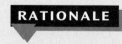

RATIONALE

This comparison helps to identify errors that may have occurred when orders were transcribed. The physician's order is the legal record of medication orders for each agency.

This knowledge aids the nurse in evaluating the therapeutic effect of the medication in relation to the patient's disorder and can also be used to educate the patient about the medication.

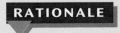

SKILL
3

Removing Medication From a Vial *(continued)*

ACTION

RATIONALE

3. Perform hand hygiene.

Hand hygiene deters the spread of microorganisms.

4. Move the medication cart to the outside of the patient's room or prepare for administration in the medication area.

Organization facilitates error-free administration and saves time.

5. Unlock the medication cart or drawer. Enter pass code and scan employee identification, if required.

Locking of the cart or drawer safeguards each patient's medication supply. Hospital accrediting organizations require medication carts to be locked when not in use. Entering pass code and scanning ID allows only authorized users into the system and identifies user for documentation by the computer.

6. **Prepare medications for one patient at a time.**

This prevents errors in medication administration.

7. Read the MAR and select the proper medication from the patient's medication drawer or unit stock.

This is the first check of the label.

8. Compare the label with the MAR. Check expiration dates and perform calculations, if necessary. Scan the bar code on the package, if required.

This is the second check of the label. Verify calculations with another nurse to ensure safety, if necessary.

9. Remove the metal or plastic cap on the vial that protects the rubber stopper.

Needs to be removed to access medication in vial.

10. **Swab the rubber top with the antimicrobial swab and allow to dry.**

Antimicrobial swab removes surface bacteria contamination. Allowing the alcohol to dry prevents it from entering the vial on the needle.

11. Remove the cap from the needle or blunt cannula by pulling it straight off. Touch the plunger at the knob only. Draw back an amount of air into the syringe that is equal to the specific dose of medication to be withdrawn. Some agencies recommend use of a filter needle when withdrawing premixed medication from multidose vials.

Before fluid is removed, injection of an equal amount of air is required to prevent the formation of a partial vacuum, because a vial is a sealed container. If not enough air is injected, the negative pressure makes it difficult to withdraw the medication. Handling plunger at knob only will keep shaft of plunger sterile. Using filter needle prevents any solid material from being withdrawn through the needle.

12. Hold the vial on a flat surface. Pierce the rubber stopper in the center with the needle tip and inject the measured air into the space above the solution (Figure 1). Do not inject air into the solution.

Air bubbled through the solution could result in withdrawal of an inaccurate amount of medication.

13. **Invert the vial. Keep the tip of the needle or blunt cannula below the fluid level (Figure 2).**

This prevents air from being aspirated into the syringe.

14. Hold the vial in one hand and use the other to withdraw the medication. Touch the plunger at the knob only. **Draw up the prescribed amount of medication while holding the syringe vertically and at eye level (Figure 3).**

Holding the syringe at eye level facilitates accurate reading, and the vertical position makes removal of air bubbles from the syringe easy. Handling plunger at knob only will keep shaft of plunger sterile.

(continued)

ACTION

RATIONALE

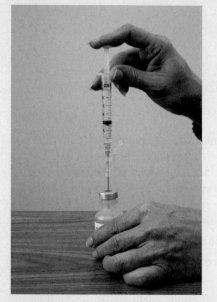

Figure 1. Injecting air with vial upright.

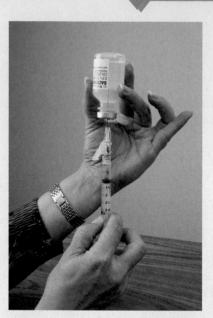

Figure 2. Positioning needle tip in solution.

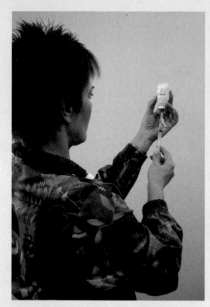

Figure 3. Withdrawing medication at eye level.

15. If any air bubbles accumulate in the syringe, tap the barrel of the syringe sharply and move the needle past the fluid into the air space to reinject the air bubble into the vial. Return the needle tip to the solution and continue withdrawal of the medication.

Removal of air bubbles is necessary to ensure accurate dose of medication.

16. After the correct dose is withdrawn, remove the needle from the vial and carefully replace the cap over the needle. If a filter needle has been used to draw up the medication, remove it and attach the appropriate administration device. Some agencies recommend changing the needle, if one was used to withdraw the medication, before administering the medication.

This prevents contamination of the needle and protects the nurse against accidental needlesticks. A one-handed recap method may be used as long as care is taken not to contaminate the needle during the process. Filter needle used to draw up medication should not be used to administer the medication to prevent any solid material from entering the patient.

17. **Check the amount of medication in the syringe with the medication dose and discard any surplus.**

Careful measurement ensures that correct dose is withdrawn.

18. **Recheck the label with the MAR.**

This is the *third* check to ensure accuracy and to prevent errors.

19. **If a multidose vial is being used, label the vial with the date and time opened, and store the vial containing the remaining medication according to agency policy.**

Because the vial is sealed, the medication inside remains sterile and can be used for future injections. Labeling the opened vials with a date and time limits its use after a specific time period.

20. Lock the medication cart before leaving it.

Locking the cart or drawer safeguards the patient's medication supply. Hospital accrediting organizations require medication carts to be locked when not in use.

21. Perform hand hygiene.

Hand hygiene deters the spread of microorganisms.

22. Proceed with administration, based on prescribed route.

See appropriate skill for prescribed route.

Removing Medication From a Vial *(continued)*

EVALUATION

The expected outcome is met when the medication is withdrawn into the syringe in a sterile manner and the proper dose is prepared.

Unexpected Situations and Associated Interventions

- *A piece of rubber stopper is noticed floating in medication in syringe:* Discard the syringe and needle and the vial. Obtain new vial and prepare dose as ordered.
- *As needle attached to syringe filled with air is inserted into vial, the plunger is immediately pulled down:* If possible to withdraw medication, continue steps as explained above. If such a vacuum has formed that this is impossible, remove syringe and inject more air into the vial. This is caused by previous withdrawal of medication without the addition of air into the vial.
- *Plunger is contaminated before injecting air into vial:* Discard needle and syringe and start over. If plunger is contaminated after medication is drawn into syringe, it is not necessary to discard and start over. The contaminated plunger will enter the barrel of the syringe when pushing the medication out and will not contaminate the medication.

SKILL VARIATION   Reconstituting Powdered Medication in a Vial

Drugs that are unstable in solution form are often provided in a dry powder form. The powder must be mixed with the correct amount of appropriate solution to prepare medication for administration. Verify the correct amount and correct solution type for the specific medication prescribed. This information is found on the vial label, package insert, in a drug reference, or from the pharmacist. To reconstitute powdered medication:

- Gather equipment. Check the medication order against the original physician's order according to agency policy.
- Know the actions, special nursing considerations, safe dose ranges, purpose of administration, and adverse effects of the medications to be administered. Consider the appropriateness of the medication for this patient.
- Perform hand hygiene.
- Move the medication cart to the outside of the patient's room or prepare for administration in the medication area
- Unlock the medication cart or drawer. Enter pass code and scan employee identification, if required.
- Prepare medications for one patient at a time.
- Read the MAR and select the proper medication and diluent from the patient's medication drawer or unit stock.
- Compare the labels with the MAR. Check expiration dates and perform calculations, if necessary. Scan the bar code on the package, if required.
- Remove the metal or plastic cap on the medication vial and diluent vial that protects the self-sealing stoppers.

- Swab the self-sealing tops with the antimicrobial swab and allow to dry.
- **Draw up the appropriate amount of diluent into the syringe.**
- Insert the needle or blunt cannula through the center of the self-sealing stopper on the powdered medication vial.
- Inject the diluent into the powdered medication vial.
- Remove the needle or blunt cannula from the vial and replace cap.
- **Gently agitate the vial to mix the powdered medication and the diluent completely. Do not shake the vial.**
- **Draw up the prescribed amount of medication while holding the syringe vertically and at eye level.**
- After the correct dose is withdrawn, remove the needle from the vial and carefully replace the cap over the needle. If a filter needle has been used to draw up the medication, remove it and attach the appropriate administration device. Some agencies recommend changing the needle, if one was used to withdraw the medication, before administering the medication.
- **Check the amount of medication in the syringe with the medication dose and discard any surplus.**
- **Recheck the label with the MAR.**
- Lock the medication cart before leaving it.
- Perform hand hygiene.
- Proceed with administration, based on prescribed route.

Mixing Medications From Two Vials in One Syringe

Preparation of medications in one syringe depends on how the medication is supplied. When using a single-dose vial and a multidose vial, air is injected into both vials and the medication in the multidose vial is drawn into the syringe first. This prevents the contents of the multidose vial from being contaminated with the medication in the single-dose vial.

When considering mixing two medications in one syringe, you must ensure that the two drugs are compatible. Nurses must be aware of drug incompatibilities when preparing medications in one syringe. Certain medications, such as diazepam (Valium), are incompatible with other drugs in the same syringe. Other drugs have limited compatibility and should be administered within 15 minutes of preparation. Incompatible drugs may become cloudy or form a precipitate in the syringe. Such medications are discarded and prepared again in separate syringes. Mixing more than two drugs in one syringe is not recommended. If it must be done, the pharmacist should be contacted to determine the compatibility of the three drugs, as well as the compatibility of their pH values and the preservatives that may be present in each drug. A drug-compatibility table should be available to nurses who are preparing medications.

Many types of insulin are available for use by patients with diabetes mellitus and are an example of medications that are often combined together in one syringe for injection, and are used as the example in the following procedure. Insulins vary in their onset and duration of action and are classified as short acting, intermediate acting, and long acting. Before administering any insulin, the nurse should be aware of the onset time, peak and duration of effects, and ensure that proper food is available. Refer to a drug reference for a listing of the different types of insulin and action specific to each type.

Insulin dosages are calculated in units. The scale commonly used is U100, which is based on 100 units of insulin contained in 1 mL of solution. Many cases of diabetes mellitus are regulated with a combination of two insulins (eg, regular and NPH insulin).

Equipment

- Two vials of medication (insulin in this example)
- Sterile syringe (insulin syringe in this example)
- Antimicrobial swabs
- Medication Administration Record (MAR) or Computer-generated MAR (CMAR)

ASSESSMENT

Determine the compatibility of the two medications. Not all insulins can be mixed together. Assess the contents of each vial of insulin. Preparations that are not modified typically appear as clear substances, so they should be without particles or foreign matter. Modified preparations are typically suspensions, so they do not appear as clear substances. It is no longer safe, however, to use the terms "clear" and "cloudy" to designate types of insulin preparation. Insulin Glargine (Lantus) is a clear but long-acting insulin (24-hour duration). It is very important to be familiar with the particular drug's properties to be able to assess the quality of the medication in the vial before withdrawal. Check expiration date before administering medication. Assess the appropriateness of the drug for the patient. Review assessment and laboratory data that may influence drug administration. Check the patient's blood glucose level if appropriate before administering the insulin. Verify patient name, dose, route, and time of administration.

NURSING DIAGNOSIS

Determine related factors for the nursing diagnoses based on the patient's current status. Appropriate nursing diagnoses include:

- Risk for Infection
- Risk for Injury
- Anxiety
- Deficient Knowledge

Mixing Medications From Two Vials in One Syringe *(continued)*

OUTCOME IDENTIFICATION AND PLANNING

The expected outcome to achieve when mixing two different types of insulin in one syringe is the accurate withdrawal of the medication into a syringe in a sterile manner and that the proper dose is prepared.

IMPLEMENTATION

ACTION	RATIONALE
1. Gather equipment. Check medication order against the original physician's order according to agency policy.	This comparison helps to identify errors that may have occurred when orders were transcribed. The physician's order is the legal record of medication orders for each agency.
2. Know the actions, special nursing considerations, safe dose ranges, purpose of administration, and adverse effects of the medications to be administered. Consider the appropriateness of the medication for this patient.	This knowledge aids the nurse in evaluating the therapeutic effect of the medication in relation to the patient's disorder and can also be used to educate the patient about the medication.
3. Perform hand hygiene.	Hand hygiene deters the spread of microorganisms.
4. Move the medication cart to the outside of the patient's room or prepare for administration in the medication area.	Organization facilitates error-free administration and saves time.
5. Unlock the medication cart or drawer. Enter pass code and scan employee identification, if required.	Locking of the cart or drawer safeguards each patient's medication supply. Hospital accrediting organizations require medication carts to be locked when not in use. Entering pass code and scanning ID allows only authorized users into the system and identifies user for documentation by the computer.
6. **Prepare medications for one patient at a time.**	This prevents errors in medication administration.
7. Read the MAR and select the proper medications from the patient's medication drawer or unit stock.	This is the first check of the labels.
8. Compare the labels with the MAR. Check expiration dates and perform calculations, if necessary. Scan the bar code on the package, if required.	This is the second check of the labels. Verify calculations with another nurse to ensure safety, if necessary.
9. If necessary, remove the cap that protects the rubber stopper on each vial.	The cap protects the rubber top.
10. **If insulin is a suspension (eg, NPH, Lente), roll and agitate the vial to mix it well.**	There is controversy regarding how to mix insulins in suspension. Some sources advise rolling the vial; others advise shaking the vial. Consult facility policy. Regardless of the method used, it is essential that the suspension be mixed well to avoid administering an inconsistent dose. Regular insulin, which is clear, does not need to be mixed before withdrawal.
11. Cleanse the rubber tops with antimicrobial swabs.	Antimicrobial swab removes surface contamination. Some sources question whether cleaning with alcohol actually disinfects or instead transfers resident bacteria from the hands to another surface.

(continued)

SKILL
4

Mixing Medications From Two Vials in One Syringe *(continued)*

ACTION

12. Remove cap from needle by pulling it straight off. Touch the plunger at the knob only. Draw back an amount of air into the syringe that is equal to the dose of modified insulin to be withdrawn.

13. Hold the modified vial on a flat surface. Pierce the rubber stopper in the center with the needle tip and inject the measured air into the space above the solution (Figure 1). Do not inject air into the solution. Withdraw the needle.

14. Draw back an amount of air into the syringe that is equal to the dose of unmodified insulin to be withdrawn.

15. Hold the unmodified vial on a flat surface. Pierce the rubber stopper in the center with the needle tip and inject the measured air into the space above the solution (Figure 2). Do not inject air into the solution. Keep the needle in the vial.

RATIONALE

Before fluid is removed, injection of an equal amount of air is required to prevent the formation of a partial vacuum, because a vial is a sealed container. If not enough air is injected, the negative pressure makes it difficult to withdraw the medication. Handling plunger by knob only ensures sterility of shaft of plunger.

Unmodified insulin should never be contaminated with modified insulin. Placing air in the modified insulin first without allowing the needle to contact the insulin ensures that the second vial entered (unmodified) insulin is not contaminated by the medication in the other vial. Air bubbled through the solution could result in withdrawal of an inaccurate amount of medication.

Before fluid is removed, injection of an equal amount of air is required to prevent the formation of a partial vacuum, because a vial is a sealed container. If not enough air is injected, the negative pressure makes it difficult to withdraw the medication.

Air bubbled through the solution could result in withdrawal of an inaccurate amount of medication.

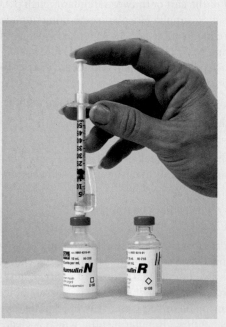

Figure 1. Injecting air into modified insulin preparation.

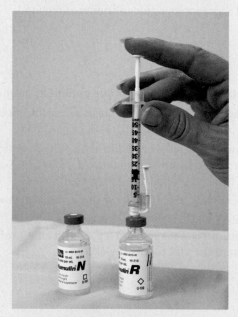

Figure 2. Injecting air into the unmodified insulin vial.

Mixing Medications From Two Vials in One Syringe *(continued)*

ACTION

16. Invert vial of unmodified insulin. Hold the vial in one hand and use the other to withdraw the medication. Touch the plunger at the knob only. **Draw up the prescribed amount of medication while holding the syringe at eye level and vertically (Figure 3).** Turn the vial over and then remove needle from vial.

17. Check that there are no air bubbles in the syringe.

18. **Check the amount of medication in the syringe with the medication dose and discard any surplus.**

19. **Recheck the vial label with the MAR.**

20. Calculate the endpoint on the syringe for the combined insulin amount by adding the number of units for each dose together.

21. Insert the needle into the modified vial and invert it, taking care not to push the plunger and inject medication from the syringe into the vial. Invert vial of modified insulin. Hold the vial in one hand and use the other to withdraw the medication. Touch the plunger at the knob only. **Draw up the prescribed amount of medication while holding the syringe at eye level and vertically (Figure 4). Take care to only withdraw the prescribed amount.** Turn the vial over and then remove needle from vial. Carefully recap the needle. Carefully replace the cap over the needle.

RATIONALE

Holding the syringe at eye level facilitates accurate reading, and the vertical position makes removal of air bubbles from the syringe easy. First dose is prepared and is not contaminated by insulin that contains modifiers.

The presence of air in the syringe would result in an inaccurate dose of medication.

Careful measurement ensures that correct dose is withdrawn.

This is the *third* check to ensure accuracy and to prevent errors.

Allows for accurate withdrawal of second dose.

Previous addition of air eliminates need to create positive pressure. Holding the syringe at eye level facilitates accurate reading. Capping the needle prevents contamination and protects the nurse against accidental needlesticks. A one-handed recap method may be used as long as care is taken to ensure that the needle remains sterile.

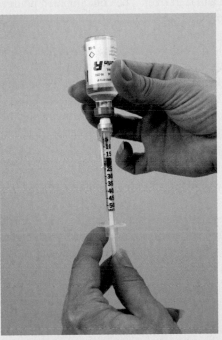

Figure 3. Withdrawing the prescribed amount of unmodified insulin.

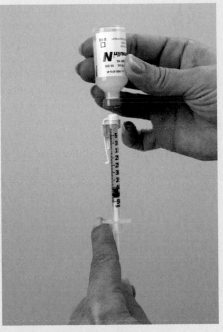

Figure 4. Withdrawing modified insulin.

(continued)

Mixing Medications From Two Vials in One Syringe *(continued)*

ACTION	RATIONALE
22. **Check the amount of medication in the syringe with the medication dose.**	Careful measurement ensures that correct dose is withdrawn.
23. **Recheck the vial label with the MAR.**	This is the *third* check to ensure accuracy and to prevent errors.
24. **Label the vials with the date and time opened, and store the vials containing the remaining medication according to agency policy.**	Because the vial is sealed, the medication inside remains sterile and can be used for future injections. Labeling the opened vials with a date and time limits its use after a specific time period.
25. Lock medication cart before leaving it.	Locking the cart or drawer safeguards the patient's medication supply. Hospital accrediting organizations require medication carts to be locked when not in use.
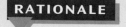 26. Perform hand hygiene.	Hand hygiene deters the spread of microorganisms.
27. Proceed with administration, based on prescribed route.	See appropriate skill for prescribed route.

EVALUATION

The expected outcome is met when the insulin is withdrawn into a syringe in a sterile manner, and the proper dose is prepared.

Unexpected Situations and Associated Interventions

- *Nurse contaminates plunger before injecting air into insulin vial:* Discard needle and syringe and start over. If plunger is contaminated after medication is drawn into the syringe, it is not necessary to discard and start over. The contaminated plunger will enter the barrel of the syringe when pushing the medication out and will not contaminate the medication.
- *Nurse allows modified insulin to come in contact with the needle before entering the unmodified insulin vial:* Discard needle and syringe and start over.
- *Nurse notices that the combined amount is not the ordered amount (eg, nurse has less or more units in combined syringe than ordered):* Discard syringe and start over. There is no way to know for sure which dosage is wrong or which medication would be expelled.
- *Nurse injects unmodified insulin into modified vial:* Discard vial and syringe and start over.

Special Considerations

General Considerations

- A diabetic patient who is visually impaired may find it helpful to use a magnifying apparatus that fits around the syringe.
- Before attempting to explain or demonstrate devices that help low-vision diabetic patients to prepare their medication, attempt to use the device yourself under similar circumstances. To detect any difficulties the patient may experience, practice using the aid with your eyes closed or in a poorly lit room.

Infant and Child Considerations

- School-age children are generally able to prepare and administer their own injections, such as insulin, with supervision (Hockenberry, 2005). Parents/significant others and the child should be involved in teaching.

Administering an Intradermal Injection

Intradermal injections are administered into the dermis, just below the epidermis. The intradermal route has the longest absorption time of all parenteral routes. For this reason, intradermal injections are used for sensitivity tests, such as tuberculin and allergy tests, and local anesthesia. The advantage of the intradermal route for these tests is that the body's reaction to substances is easily visible, and degrees of reaction are discernible by comparative study.

Sites commonly used are the inner surface of the forearm and the upper back, under the scapula. Equipment used for an intradermal injection includes a tuberculin syringe calibrated in tenths and hundredths of a milliliter and a ¼″ to ½″, 26- or 27-gauge needle. The dosage given intradermally is small, usually less than 0.5 mL. The angle of administration for an intradermal injection is 10–15 degrees.

Equipment

- Prescribed medication
- Sterile syringe, usually a tuberculin syringe calibrated in tenths and hundredths, and needle, ¼″ to ½″, 26- or 27-gauge
- Antimicrobial swab
- Disposable gloves
- Small gauze square
- Medication Administration Record (MAR) or Computer-generated MAR (CMAR)

ASSESSMENT

Assess the patient for any allergies. Check expiration date before administering medication. Assess the appropriateness of the drug for the patient. Review assessment and laboratory data that may influence drug administration. Assess the site on the patient where the injection is to be given. Avoid areas of broken or open skin. Avoid areas that are highly pigmented, have lesions, bruises, or scars and are hairy. Assess the patient's knowledge of the medication. This may provide an opportune time for patient education. Verify the patient's name, dose, route, and time of administration.

NURSING DIAGNOSIS

Determine related factors for the nursing diagnoses based on the patient's current status. Appropriate nursing diagnoses may include:

- Deficient Knowledge
- Risk for Allergy Response
- Risk for Infection
- Risk for Injury
- Anxiety

OUTCOME IDENTIFICATION AND PLANNING

The expected outcome to achieve when administering an intradermal injection is appearance of a wheal at the site of injection. Other outcomes that may be appropriate include the following: the patient refrains from rubbing the site; the patient's anxiety is decreased; the patient does not experience adverse effects; and the patient understands and complies with the medication regimen.

IMPLEMENTATION

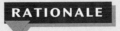

ACTION	RATIONALE
1. Gather equipment. Check each medication order against the original physician's order according to agency policy. Clarify any inconsistencies. Check the patient's chart for allergies.	This comparison helps to identify errors that may have occurred when orders were transcribed. The physician's order is the legal record of medication orders for each agency.

(continued)

Administering an Intradermal Injection *(continued)*

ACTION	RATIONALE
2. Know the actions, special nursing considerations, safe dose ranges, purpose of administration, and adverse effects of the medications to be administered. Consider the appropriateness of the medication for this patient.	This knowledge aids the nurse in evaluating the therapeutic effect of the medication in relation to the patient's disorder and can also be used to educate the patient about the medication.
3. Perform hand hygiene.	Hand hygiene prevents the spread of microorganisms.
4. Move the medication cart to the outside of the patient's room or prepare for administration in the medication area.	Organization facilitates error-free administration and saves time.
5. Unlock the medication cart or drawer. Enter pass code and scan employee identification, if required.	Locking of the cart or drawer safeguards each patient's medication supply. Hospital accrediting organizations require medication carts to be locked when not in use. Entering pass code and scanning ID allows only authorized users into the system and identifies user for documentation by the computer.
6. **Prepare medications for one patient at a time.**	This prevents errors in medication administration.
7. Read the MAR and select the proper medication from the patient's medication drawer or unit stock.	This is the first check of the label.
8. Compare the label with the MAR. Check expiration dates and perform calculations, if necessary. Scan the bar code on the package, if required.	This is the second check of the label. Verify calculations with another nurse to ensure safety, if necessary.
9. If necessary, withdraw medication from an ampule or vial as described in Skills 2 and 3.	
10. **When all medications for one patient have been prepared, recheck the label with the MAR before taking them to the patient.**	This is a *third* check to ensure accuracy and to prevent errors.
11. Lock the medication cart before leaving it.	Locking the cart or drawer safeguards the patient's medication supply. Hospital accrediting organizations require medication carts to be locked when not in use.
12. Transport medications to the patient's bedside carefully, and keep the medications in sight at all times.	Careful handling and close observation prevent accidental or deliberate disarrangement of medications.
13. **Ensure that the patient receives the medications at the correct time.**	Check agency policy, which may allow for administration within a period of 30 minutes before or 30 minutes after designated time.
14. **Identify the patient.** Usually, the patient should be identified using two methods. Compare information with the MAR or CMAR.	Identifying the patient ensures the right patient receives the medications and helps prevent errors.
a. Check the name and identification number on the patient's identification band.	This is the most reliable method. Replace the identification band if it is missing or inaccurate in any way.
b. Ask the patient to state his or her name.	This requires a response from the patient, but illness and strange surroundings often cause patients to be confused.
c. If the patient cannot identify him or herself, verify the patient's identification with a staff member who knows the patient for the second source.	This is another way to double-check identity. Do not use the name on the door or over the bed, because these may be inaccurate.

Administering an Intradermal Injection *(continued)*

ACTION

RATIONALE

15. Close the door to the room or pull the bedside curtain.

This provides patient privacy.

16. Complete necessary assessments before administering medications. Check allergy bracelet or ask patient about allergies. Explain the purpose and action of the medication to the patient.

Assessment is a prerequisite to administration of medications. Explanation provides rationale, increases knowledge, and reduces anxiety.

17. Scan the patient's bar code on the identification band, if required.

Provides additional check to ensure that the medication is given to the right patient.

18. Perform hand hygiene and put on clean gloves.

Hand hygiene prevents the spread of microorganisms. Gloves help prevent exposure to contaminants.

19. Select an appropriate administration site. Assist the patient to the appropriate position for the site chosen. Drape as needed to expose only area of site to be used.

Appropriate site prevents injury and allows for accurate reading of the test site at the appropriate time.

20. Cleanse the site with an antimicrobial swab while wiping with a firm, circular motion and moving outward from the injection site. Allow the skin to dry.

Pathogens on the skin can be forced into the tissues by the needle. Moving from the center outward prevents contamination of the site. Allowing skin to dry prevents introducing alcohol into the tissue, which can be irritating and uncomfortable.

21. Remove the needle cap with the nondominant hand by pulling it straight off.

This technique lessens the risk of an accidental needlestick.

22. Use the nondominant hand to spread the skin taut over the injection site (Figure 1).

Taut skin provides an easy entrance into intradermal tissue.

23. Hold the syringe in the dominant hand, between the thumb and forefinger with the bevel of the needle up.

Using dominant hand allows for easy, appropriate handling of syringe. Having the bevel up allows for smooth piercing of the skin and introduction of medication into the dermis.

24. Hold the syringe at a 10 to 15 degree angle from the site. **Place the needle almost flat against the patient's skin (Figure 2), bevel side up, and insert the needle into the skin so that the point of the needle can be seen through the skin. Insert the needle only about ⅛″ with entire bevel under the skin.**

The dermis is entered when the needle is held as nearly parallel to the skin as possible and is inserted about ⅛″.

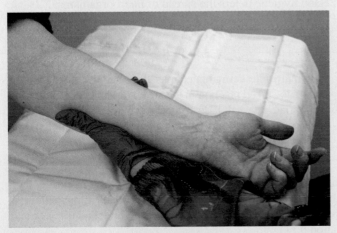

Figure 1. Spreading the skin taut over the injection site.

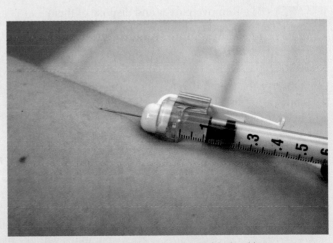

Figure 2. Inserting the needle almost level with the skin.

(continued)

Administering an Intradermal Injection *(continued)*

ACTION

RATIONALE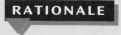

25. Once the needle is in place, steady the lower end of the syringe. Slide your dominant hand to the end of the plunger.

Prevents injury and inadvertent advancement or withdrawal of needle.

26. Slowly inject the agent while watching for a small wheal or blister to appear (Figure 3).

The appearance of a wheal indicates the medication is in the dermis.

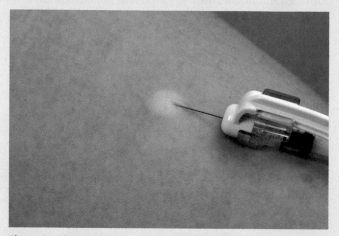

Figure 3. Observing for wheal while injecting medication.

27. Withdraw the needle quickly at the same angle that it was inserted.

Withdrawing the needle quickly and at the angle at which it entered the skin minimizes tissue damage and discomfort for the patient.

28. **Do not massage area after removing needle. Tell patient not to rub or scratch site. If necessary, gently blot the site with a dry gauze square. Do not apply pressure or rub the site.**

Massaging the area where an intradermal injection is given may spread the medication to underlying subcutaneous tissue.

29. Do not recap the used needle. Engage the safety shield or needle guard, if present. Discard the needle and syringe in the appropriate receptacle.

Proper disposal of the needle prevents injury.

30. Assist the patient to a position of comfort.

This provides for the well-being of the patient.

 31. Remove gloves and dispose of them properly. Perform hand hygiene.

Hand hygiene deters the spread of microorganisms.

32. Observe the area for signs of a reaction at determined intervals after administration. Inform the patient of the need for inspection.

With many intradermal injections, the nurse will need to look for a localized reaction in the area of the injection at the appropriate interval(s) determined by the type of medication and purpose. Preparing the patient increases compliance.

EVALUATION

The expected outcomes are met when the nurse notes a wheal at site of injection; the patient refrains from rubbing the site; the patient's anxiety is decreased; the patient did not experience adverse effects; and the patient verbalizes an understanding of and complies with the medication regimen.

SKILL 5   Administering an Intradermal Injection *(continued)*

DOCUMENTATION

Guidelines

Record each medication given on the MAR or record using the required format, including date, time, and the site of administration, immediately after administration. Some agencies recommend circling the injection site with ink (Figure 4). Circling the injection site easily identifies the site of the intradermal injection and allows for careful observation of the exact area. If using a bar-code system, medication administration is automatically recorded when scanned. PRN medications require documentation of the reason for administration. Prompt recording avoids the possibility of accidentally repeating the administration of the drug. If the drug was refused or omitted, record this in the appropriate area on the medication record and notify the physician. This verifies the reason medication was omitted and ensures that the physician is aware of the patient's condition.

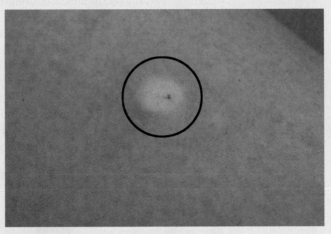

Figure 4. Drawing a circle around the wheal on skin.

Unexpected Situations and Associated Interventions

- *Nurse does not note wheal or blister at site of injection:* Medication has been injected subcutaneously. Document according to facility policy and inform the physician. Nurse may need to obtain order to repeat procedure.
- *Medication leaks out of injection site before needle is withdrawn:* Needle was inserted less than ⅛″. Document according to facility policy and inform the physician. Nurse may need to obtain order to repeat procedure.
- *Nurse sticks self with needle before injection:* Discard needle and syringe appropriately. Follow agency policy regarding needlestick injury. Prepare new syringe with medication and administer to patient. Complete appropriate paperwork and follow agency's policy regarding accidental needlesticks.
- *Nurse sticks self with needle after injection:* Discard needle and syringe appropriately. Follow agency policy regarding needlestick injury. Complete appropriate paperwork and follow agency's policy regarding accidental needlesticks.

Special Considerations

General Considerations

- Ongoing assessment is an important part of nursing care to evaluate patient response to administered medications and early detection of adverse effects. If an adverse effect is suspected, withhold further medication doses and notify the patient's primary healthcare provider. Additional intervention is based on type of reaction and patient assessment.
- Aspiration, pulling back on the plunger after insertion and before administration, is not recommended for an intradermal injection. The dermis does not contain large blood vessels.
- Some agencies recommend administering intradermal injections with the bevel down instead of the bevel up. Check facility policy.

Administering a Subcutaneous Injection

Subcutaneous injections are administered into the adipose tissue layer just below the epidermis and dermis. This tissue has few blood vessels, so drugs administered here have a slow, sustained rate of absorption into the capillaries.

To correctly and effectively administer a subcutaneous injection, the nurse must choose the right equipment, select the appropriate location, use the correct technique, and deliver the correct dose.

It is important to choose the right equipment to ensure depositing the medication into the intended tissue layer and not the underlying muscle. Equipment used for a subcutaneous injection includes a syringe of appropriate volume for the amount of drug being administered. (An insulin pen may be used for subcutaneous injection of insulin; see the accompanying Skill Variation for technique). A 25-to 30-gauge, ⅜″ to 1″ needle can be used. The ⅜″ and ⅝″ needles are most commonly used. Some medications are packaged in prefilled cartridges with a needle attached. Confirm that the provided needle is appropriate for the patient before use. If not, the medication will have to be transferred to another syringe and the appropriate needle attached. Review the specifics of the particular medication before administrating. Various sites may be used for subcutaneous injections, including the outer aspect of the upper arm, the abdomen (from below the costal margin to the iliac crests), the anterior aspects of the thigh, the upper back, and the upper ventral or dorsogluteal area. Figure 1 shows the sites on the body where subcutaneous injections can be given. Absorption rates are different from the different sites. Injections in the abdomen are most rapidly absorbed, somewhat slower from the arms, even slower from the thighs, and slowest from the upper ventral or dorsogluteal areas (Caffrey, 2003).

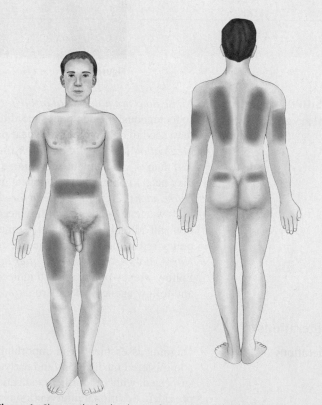

Figure 1. Sites on the body where subcutaneous injections can be given.

Administering a Subcutaneous Injection (continued)

Subcutaneous injections are administered at a 45–90 degree angle. Choose the angle of needle insertion based on the amount of subcutaneous tissue present and the length of the needle. Generally, the shorter, ⅜″ needle should be inserted at a 90-degree angle and the longer, ⅝″ needle is inserted at a 45-degree angle.

Recommendations differ regarding pinching or bunching of a skin fold for administration. Pinching is advised for thinner patients and when a longer needle is used, to lift the adipose tissue away from underlying muscle and tissue. If pinching is used, once the needle is inserted, release the skin to avoid injecting into compressed tissue (King, 2003; Rushing, 2004; Stephens, 2003a).

Aspiration, or pulling back on the plunger to check that a blood vessel has been entered, is not necessary and has not proved to be a reliable indicator of needle placement. The likelihood of injecting into a blood vessel is small (Rushing, 2004; Stephens, 2003b). Aspiration is definitely contraindicated with administration of heparin because this action can result in hematoma formation.

Usually, no more than 1 mL of solution is given subcutaneously. Giving larger amounts adds to the patient's discomfort and may predispose to poor absorption

Equipment

- Prescribed medication
- Sterile syringe and needle. Needle size depends on the medication administered and patient body type (see previous discussion).
- Antimicrobial swab
- Disposable gloves
- Small gauze square
- Medication Administration Record (MAR) or Computer-generated MAR (CMAR)

ASSESSMENT

Assess the patient for any allergies. Check expiration date before administering medication. Assess the appropriateness of the drug for the patient. Verify patient name, dose, route, and time of administration. Review assessment and laboratory data that may influence drug administration. Assess the site on the patient where the injection is to be given. Avoid sites that are bruised, tender, hard, swollen, inflamed, or scarred. These conditions could affect absorption or cause discomfort and injury (Rushing, 2004). Assess the patient's knowledge of the medication. If the patient has deficient knowledge about the medication, this may be the appropriate time to begin education about the medication. If the medication may affect the patient's vital signs, assess them before administration. If the medication is for pain relief, assess the patient's pain level before and after administration.

NURSING DIAGNOSIS

Determine related factors for the nursing diagnoses based on the patient's current status. Appropriate nursing diagnoses may include:

- Deficient Knowledge
- Acute Pain
- Risk for Infection
- Risk for Injury
- Anxiety
- Risk for Allergy Response

OUTCOME IDENTIFICATION AND PLANNING

The expected outcome is that the patient receives medication via the subcutaneous route. Other outcomes that may be appropriate include the following: the patient's anxiety is decreased; the patient does not experience adverse effects; and the patient understands and complies with the medication regimen.

(continued)

SKILL
6

Administering a Subcutaneous Injection *(continued)*

IMPLEMENTATION

ACTION

RATIONALE

1. Gather equipment. Check each medication order against the original physician's order according to agency policy. Clarify any inconsistencies. Check the patient's chart for allergies.

   This comparison helps to identify errors that may have occurred when orders were transcribed. The physician's order is the legal record of medication orders for each agency.

2. Know the actions, special nursing considerations, safe dose ranges, purpose of administration, and adverse effects of the medications to be administered. Consider the appropriateness of the medication for this patient.

   This knowledge aids the nurse in evaluating the therapeutic effect of the medication in relation to the patient's disorder and can also be used to educate the patient about the medication.

 3. Perform hand hygiene.

   Hand hygiene prevents the spread of microorganisms.

4. Move the medication cart to the outside of the patient's room or prepare for administration in the medication area.

   Organization facilitates error-free administration and saves time.

5. Unlock the medication cart or drawer. Enter pass code and scan employee identification, if required.

   Locking of the cart or drawer safeguards each patient's medication supply. Hospital accrediting organizations require medication carts to be locked when not in use. Entering pass code and scanning ID allows only authorized users into the system and identifies user for documentation by the computer.

6. **Prepare medications for one patient at a time.**

   This prevents errors in medication administration.

7. Read the MAR and select the proper medication from the patient's medication drawer or unit stock.

   This is the first check of the label.

8. Compare the label with the MAR. Check expiration dates and perform calculations, if necessary. Scan the bar code on the package, if required.

   This is the second check of the label. Verify calculations with another nurse to ensure safety, if necessary.

9. If necessary, withdraw medication from an ampule or vial as described in Skills 2 and 3.

10. **When all medications for one patient have been prepared, recheck the label with the MAR before taking them to the patient.**

    This is a *third* check to ensure accuracy and to prevent errors.

11. Lock the medication cart before leaving it.

    Locking the cart or drawer safeguards the patient's medication supply. Hospital accrediting organizations require medication carts to be locked when not in use.

12. Transport medications to the patient's bedside carefully, and keep the medications in sight at all times.

    Careful handling and close observation prevent accidental or deliberate disarrangement of medications.

13. **Ensure that the patient receives the medications at the correct time.**

    Check agency policy, which may allow for administration within a period of 30 minutes before or 30 minutes after designated time.

ACTION	RATIONALE

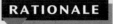

14. **Identify the patient.** Usually, the patient should be identified using two methods. Compare information with the MAR or CMAR.

Identifying the patient ensures the right patient receives the medications and helps prevent errors.

a. Check the name and identification number on the patient's identification band.

This is the most reliable method. Replace the identification band if it is missing or inaccurate in any way.

b. Ask the patient to state his or her name.

This requires a response from the patient, but illness and strange surroundings often cause patients to be confused.

c. If the patient cannot identify him or herself, verify the patient's identification with a staff member who knows the patient for the second source.

This is another way to double-check identity. Do not use the name on the door or over the bed, because these may be inaccurate.

15. Close the door to the room or pull the bedside curtain.

This provides patient privacy.

16. Complete necessary assessments before administering medications. Check allergy bracelet or ask patient about allergics. Explain the purpose and action of the medication to the patient.

Assessment is a prerequisite to administration of medications. Explanation provides rationale, increases knowledge, and reduces anxiety.

17. Scan the patient's bar code on the identification band, if required.

Scanning provides additional check to ensure that the medication is given to the right patient.

18. Perform hand hygiene and put on clean gloves.

Hand hygiene prevents the spread of microorganisms. Gloves help prevent exposure to contaminants.

19. Select an appropriate administration site.

Appropriate site prevents injury and allows for accurate reading of the test site at the appropriate time.

20. Assist the patient to the appropriate position for the site chosen. Drape as needed to expose only area of site to be used.

Draping helps maintain the patient's privacy.

21. Identify the appropriate landmarks for the site chosen.

Good visualization is necessary to establish the correct location of the site and to avoid damage to tissues.

22. Clean the area around the injection site with an anti-microbial swab. Use a firm, circular motion while moving outward from the injection site (Figure 2). Allow area to dry.

Pathogens on the skin can be forced into the tissues by the needle. Moving from the center outward prevents contamination of the site. Allowing skin to dry prevents introducing alcohol into the tissue, which can be irritating and uncomfortable.

23. Remove the needle cap with the nondominant hand, pulling it straight off.

The cap protects the needle from contact with micro-organisms. This technique lessens the risk of an accidental needlestick.

24. Grasp and bunch the area surrounding the injection site or spread the skin taut at the site (Figure 3).

Decision to create a skin fold is based on the nurse's assessment of the patient and needle length used. Pinching is advised for thinner patients and when a longer needle is used, to lift the adipose tissue away from underlying muscle and tissue. If pinching is used, once the needle is inserted, release the skin to avoid injecting into compressed tissue. If skin is pulled taut, it provides easy, less painful entry into the subcutaneous tissue.

(continued)

Administering a Subcutaneous Injection (continued)

ACTION

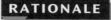
RATIONALE

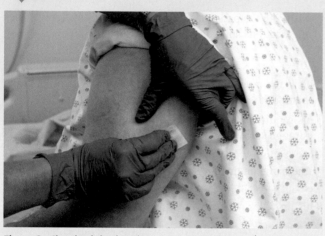

Figure 2. Cleaning injection site.

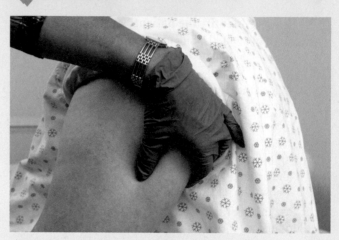

Figure 3. Bunching tissue around injection site.

25. **Hold the syringe in the dominant hand between the thumb and forefinger. Inject the needle quickly at a 45–90 degree angle (Figure 4).**

26. After the needle is in place, release the tissue. If you have a large skin fold pinched up, ensure that the needle stays in place as the skin is released. Immediately move your nondominant hand to steady the lower end of the syringe. Slide your dominant hand to the end of the plunger. Avoid moving the syringe.

27. Inject the medication slowly (at a rate of 10 seconds per milliliter).

28. Withdraw the needle quickly at the same angle at which it was inserted, while supporting the surrounding tissue with your nondominant hand (Figure 5).

Inserting the needle quickly causes less pain to the patient. Subcutaneous tissue is abundant in well-nourished, well-hydrated people and spare in emaciated, dehydrated, or very thin persons. For a person with little subcutaneous tissue, it is best to insert the needle at a 45-degree angle.

Injecting the solution into compressed tissues results in pressure against nerve fibers and creates discomfort. If there is a large skin fold, the skin may retract away from the needle. The nondominant hand secures the syringe. Moving the syringe could cause damage to the tissues and inadvertent administration into incorrect area.

Rapid injection of the solution creates pressure in the tissues, resulting in discomfort.

Slow withdrawal of the needle pulls the tissues and causes discomfort. Applying counter traction around the injection site helps to prevent pulling on the tissue as the needle is withdrawn. Removing the needle at the same angle at which it was inserted minimizes tissue damage and discomfort for the patient.

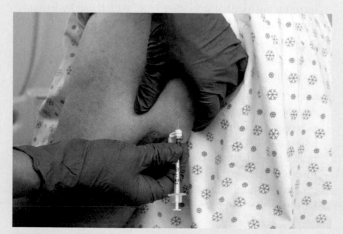

Figure 4. Inserting needle.

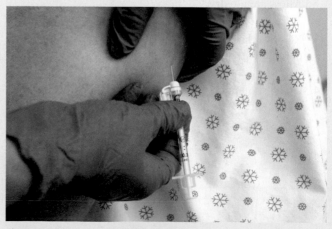

Figure 5. Withdrawing needle.

SKILL
6

Administering a Subcutaneous Injection *(continued)*

ACTION	RATIONALE

29. **Using a gauze square, apply gentle pressure to the site after the needle is withdrawn (Figure 6). Do not massage the site.**

Massaging the site is not necessary and can damage underlying tissue and increase the absorption of the medication. Massaging after heparin administration can contribute to hematoma formation. Massaging after an insulin injection may contribute to unpredictable absorption of the medication.

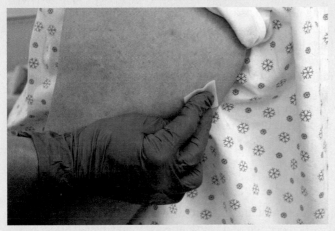

Figure 6. Applying pressure to the injection site.

30. Do not recap the used needle. Engage the safety shield or needle guard, if present. Discard the needle and syringe in the appropriate receptacle.

Proper disposal of the needle prevents injury.

31. Assist the patient to a position of comfort.

This provides for the well-being of the patient.

32. Remove gloves and dispose of them properly. Perform hand hygiene.

Hand hygiene deters the spread of microorganisms.

33. Evaluate the response of the patient to the medication within an appropriate time frame for the particular medication.

Evaluate effectiveness of drug and provides early detection of adverse effect.

EVALUATION

The expected outcomes are met when the patient receives the medication via the subcutaneous route; the patient's anxiety is decreased; the patient does not experience adverse effects; and the patient understands and complies with the medication regimen.

DOCUMENTATION

Guidelines

Record each medication given on the MAR or record using the required format, including date, dose, time, and the site of administration, immediately after administration. If using a bar-code system, medication administration is automatically recorded when scanned. PRN medications require documentation of the reason for administration. Prompt recording avoids the possibility of accidentally repeating the administration of the drug. If the drug was refused or omitted, record this in the appropriate area on the medication record and notify the physician. This verifies the reason medication was omitted and ensures that the physician is aware of the patient's condition.

(continued)

Unexpected Situations and Associated Interventions

- *When skin fold is released, needle pulls out of skin:* Remove and appropriately discard needle. Attach new needle to syringe and administer injection.
- *Patient refuses to let nurse administer medication in a different location:* Explain the rationale behind rotating injection sites. Discuss other available injection sites with patient. If patient will still not allow injection in another area, administer medication to patient, document patient's refusal and discussion, and notify physician.
- *Nurse sticks self with needle before injection:* Discard needle and syringe appropriately. Follow agency policy regarding needlestick injury. Prepare new syringe with medication and administer to patient. Complete appropriate paperwork and follow agency's policy regarding accidental needlesticks.
- *Nurse sticks self with needle after injection:* Discard needle and syringe appropriately. Follow agency policy regarding needlestick injury. Complete appropriate paperwork and follow agency's policy regarding accidental needlesticks.
- *During injection, patient pulls away from needle before medication is delivered fully:* Remove and appropriately discard needle. Attach a new needle to syringe and administer remaining medication at a different site. Document events and interventions according to facility policy.

Special Considerations

General Considerations

Ongoing assessment is an important part of nursing care to evaluate patient response to administered medications and early detection of adverse effects. If an adverse effect is suspected, withhold further medication doses and notify the patient's primary healthcare provider. Additional intervention is based on type of reaction and patient assessment.

Infant and Child Considerations

- Do not tell a child that an injection will not hurt. Describe the feel of the injection as a pinch or a sting. A child who believes you have been dishonest with him or her is less likely to cooperate with future procedures.

Older Adult Considerations

- Many elderly patients have less adipose tissue. Adjust the angle of the needle and angle of insertion accordingly. You do not want to inadvertently give a subcutaneous medication intramuscularly.

Home Care Considerations

- Reuse of syringes in the home setting is not recommended. Changes and improvements to insulin syringes to make injections painless have resulted in thinner, shorter, sharper, and better lubricated needles. As a result, after one injection the tip of the fine needles can bend and form a hook that can tear tissue if reused. These fine needles can break and leave fragments in the skin and tissue if reused. Reuse results in more painful injections related to a reduction in needle lubricant and tip damage (Caffrey, 2003; King, 2003).
- Encourage patients to consult the policies of their local government regarding contaminated and sharps waste disposal. Needles and syringes should be disposed of in a hard, plastic container. Liquid detergent or liquid fabric softener containers are good choices. Glass containers should not be used.

SKILL
6

Administering a Subcutaneous Injection *(continued)*

SKILL VARIATION **Using an Insulin Pen to Administer Insulin via the Subcutaneous Route**

- Perform hand hygiene.
- Remove the pen cap.
- Insert an insulin cartridge into the pen, following the manufacturer's directions.
- Clean the tip of the reservoir with alcohol.
- Invert the pen 20 times to mix if using an insulin suspension.
- Remove the protective tab from the needle.
- Screw the needle onto the reservoir.
- Remove the outer and inner needle caps.
- Hold the pen upright and tap to force any air bubbles to the top.
- Dial the dose selector to 2 units to perform an "air shot" to get rid of bubbles.

- Hold the pen upright and press the plunger firmly. Watch for a drop of insulin at the needle tip.
- Check the drug reservoir to make sure enough insulin is available for the dose.
- Check that the dose selector is at "0," and then dial the units of insulin for the dose.
- Clean the injection site and administer the subcutaneous injection, holding the pen like a dart. Push the button on the pen all the way in.
- Keep the button depressed and count to 6 before removing from the skin.
- Remove the needle from the pen and dispose in a sharps container. Perform hand hygiene.

(Adapted from Moshang, J. [2005]. Making a point about insulin pens. *Nursing, 35*[2], 46–47.)

SKILL
7

Administering an Intramuscular Injection

Intramuscular injections deliver medication through the skin and subcutaneous tissues into certain muscles. Muscles have larger and a greater number of blood vessels than subcutaneous tissue, allowing faster onset of action than with subcutaneous injections. Some medications administered intramuscularly are formulated to have a longer duration of effect. The deposit of medication creates a depot at the site of injection, designed to deliver slow, sustained release over hours, days, or weeks.

To correctly and effectively administer an intramuscular injection, the nurse must choose the right equipment, select the appropriate location, use the correct technique, and deliver the correct dose.

It is important to choose the right needle length for a particular intramuscular injection. Needle length should be based on the site for injection and the patient's age. See Table 5

TABLE 1 **Intramuscular Injection Needle Length**	
SITE/AGE	**NEEDLE LENGTH**
Vastus lateralis	⅝" to 1"
Deltoid (children)	⅝" to 1¼"
Deltoid (adults)	1" to 1½"
Ventrogluteal (adults)	1½"

(Adapted from Nicoll, L. & Hesby, A. [2002]. Intramuscular injection: An integrative research review and guideline for evidence-based practice. *Applied Nursing Research, 16*[2], 149–162.)

(continued)

Administering an Intramuscular Injection (continued)

for intramuscular needle length recommendations. Patients who are obese may require a longer needle, and emaciated patients may require a shorter needle. Appropriate gauge is determined by the medication being administered. Generally, biologic agents and medications in aqueous solutions should be administered with a 20-to 25-gauge needle. Medications in oil-based solutions should be administered with an 18-to 25-gauge needle. Many medications come in prefilled syringe units. If a needle is provided on the prefilled unit, the nurse should ensure that the needle on the unit is the appropriate length for the patient and situation.

To avoid complications, the nurse must be able to identify anatomic landmarks and site boundaries. The age of the patient, medication type, and medication volume should

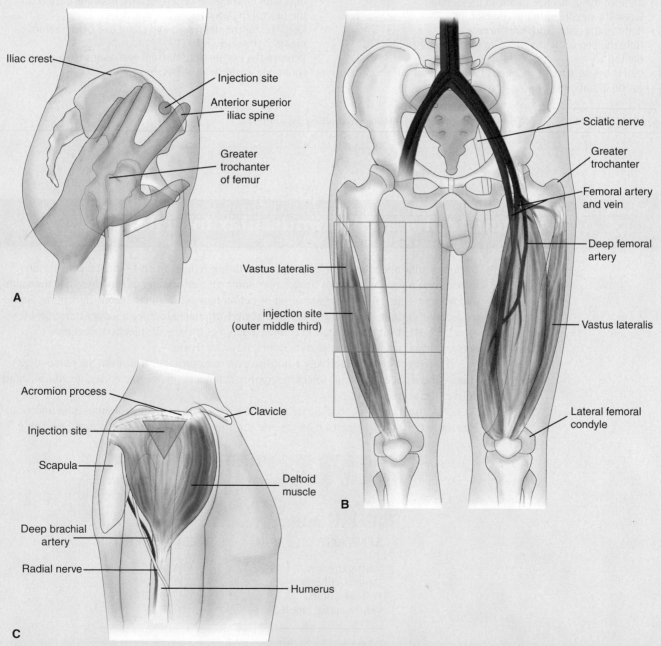

Figure 1. Sites for intramuscular injections. Descriptions for locating the sites are given in the text. (**A**) The ventrogluteal site is located by placing the palm on the greater trochanter and the index finger toward the anterosuperior iliac spine. (**B**) The vastus lateralis site is identified by dividing the thigh into thirds, horizontally and vertically. (**C**) The deltoid muscle site is located by palpating the lower edge of the acromion process.

Administering an Intramuscular Injection *(continued)*

be considered when selecting a site for intramuscular injection. See Table 2 for information related to intramuscular site selection. The sites used to administer intramuscular medications should be rotated when therapy requires repeated injections. Whatever pattern of rotating sites is used, a description of it should appear in the patient's plan of nursing care. Depending on the site selected, the nurse may need to reposition the patient (see Table 3).

The nurse should use accurate, careful technique when administering intramuscular injections. If care is not taken, possible complications include abscesses, cellulites, injury to blood vessels, bones and nerves, lingering pain, tissue necrosis, and periostitis (inflammation of the membrane covering a bone). Administer the intramuscular injection so that the needle is perpendicular to the patient's body. This ensures it is given using an angle of injection between 72 to 90 degrees (Nicoll & Hesby, 2002).

TABLE 2 Intramuscular Site Selection

	RECOMMENDED SITE
Age of Patient	
Infants	Vastus lateralis
Toddlers and children	Vastus lateralis or deltoid
Adults	Ventrogluteal or deltoid
Medication Type	
Biologicals (infants and young children)	Vastus lateralis
Biologicals (older children and adults)	Deltoid
Hepatitis B/Rabies	Deltoid
Depot formulations	Ventrogluteal
Medications that are known to be irritating, viscous, or oily solutions	Ventrogluteal

(Adapted from Nicoll, L. & Hesby, A. [2002]. Intramuscular injection: An integrative research review and guideline for evidence-based practice. *Applied Nursing Research, 16*[2], 149–162.)

TABLE 3 Patient Positioning

SITE OF INJECTION	PATIENT POSITION
Deltoid	Patient may sit or stand. A child may be held in an adult's lap.
Ventrogluteal	Patient may stand, sit, lay laterally, lay supine.
Vastus lateralis	Patient may sit or lay supine. Infants and young children may lay supine or be held in an adult's lap.

(Adapted from Nicoll, L. & Hesby, A. [2002]. Intramuscular injection: An integrative research review and guideline for evidence-based practice. *Applied Nursing Research, 16*[2], 149–162.)

The volume of medication that can be administered intramuscularly varies based on the intended site. Generally, 1 to 4 mL is the accepted volume range, with no more than 1 to 2 mL given at the deltoid site. The less-developed muscles of children and elderly people limit the intramuscular injection to 1 to 2 mL.

(continued)

Equipment

- Disposable gloves
- Medication
- Sterile syringe and needle of appropriate size and gauge
- Antimicrobial swab
- Small gauze square
- Medication Administration Record (MAR) or Computer-generated MAR (CMAR)

ASSESSMENT

Assess the patient's knowledge of the medication. If the patient has a knowledge deficit about the medication, this may be an appropriate time to begin education about the medication. Assess the area where the injection is to be given. If the medication is for pain, assess the patient's level of pain. If the medication may affect the patient's vital signs or laboratory test results, check them before administering the medication. Assess the patient for any allergies. Check expiration date before administering medication. Assess the appropriateness of the drug for the patient. Verify patient name, medication dose, route, and time of administration. Review assessment and laboratory data that may influence drug administration. Assess the site on the patient where the injection is to be given. Avoid any site that is bruised, tender, hard, swollen, inflamed, or scarred. Assess the patient's knowledge of the medication. If the patient has a knowledge deficit about the medication, this may be the appropriate time to begin education about the medication. If the medication may affect the patient's vital signs, assess them before administration. If the medication is for pain relief, assess the patient's pain level before and after administration

NURSING DIAGNOSIS

Determine related factors for the nursing diagnoses based on the patient's current status. Appropriate diagnoses may include:

- Deficient Knowledge
- Acute Pain
- Risk for Allergy Response
- Anxiety
- Risk for Injury
- Risk for Impaired Skin Integrity

OUTCOME IDENTIFICATION AND PLANNING

The expected outcome to achieve when administering an intramuscular injection is that the patient receives the medication via the intramuscular route. Other outcomes that may be appropriate include the following: the patient's anxiety is decreased; the patient does not experience adverse effects; and the patient understands and complies with the medication regimen.

IMPLEMENTATION

ACTION

1. Gather equipment. Check each medication order against the original physician's order according to agency policy. Clarify any inconsistencies. Check the patient's chart for allergies.

2. Know the actions, special nursing considerations, safe dose ranges, purpose of administration, and adverse effects of the medications to be administered. Consider the appropriateness of the medication for this patient.

RATIONALE

This comparison helps to identify errors that may have occurred when orders were transcribed. The physician's order is the legal record of medication orders for each agency.

This knowledge aids the nurse in evaluating the therapeutic effect of the medication in relation to the patient's disorder and can also be used to educate the patient about the medication.

Administering an Intramuscular Injection *(continued)*

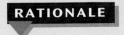

ACTION

3. Perform hand hygiene.

4. Move the medication cart to the outside of the patient's room or prepare for administration in the medication area.

5. Unlock the medication cart or drawer. Enter pass code and scan employee identification, if required.

6. **Prepare medications for one patient at a time.**

7. Read the MAR and select the proper medication from the patient's medication drawer or unit stock.

8. Compare the label with the MAR. Check expiration dates and perform calculations, if necessary. Scan the bar code on the package, if required.

9. If necessary, withdraw medication from an ampule or vial as described in Skills 2 and 3.

10. **When all medications for one patient have been prepared, recheck the label with the MAR before taking them to the patient.**

11. Lock the medication cart before leaving it.

12. Transport medications to the patient's bedside carefully, and keep the medications in sight at all times.

13. **Ensure that the patient receives the medications at the correct time.**

14. **Identify the patient.** Usually, the patient should be identified using two methods. Compare information with the MAR or CMAR.

    a. Check the name and identification number on the patient's identification band.

    b. Ask the patient to state his or her name.

    c. If the patient cannot identify him or herself, verify the patient's identification with a staff member who knows the patient for the second source.

15. Close the door to the room or pull the bedside curtain.

16. Complete necessary assessments before administering medications. Check allergy bracelet or ask patient about allergies. Explain the purpose and action of the medication to the patient.

RATIONALE

Hand hygiene prevents the spread of microorganisms.

Organization facilitates error-free administration and saves time.

Locking of the cart or drawer safeguards each patient's medication supply. Hospital accrediting organizations require medication carts to be locked when not in use. Entering pass code and scanning ID allows only authorized users into the system and identifies user for documentation by the computer.

This prevents errors in medication administration.

This is the first check of the label.

This is the second check of the label. Verify calculations with another nurse to ensure safety, if necessary.

This is a *third* check to ensure accuracy and to prevent errors.

Locking the cart or drawer safeguards the patient's medication supply. Hospital accrediting organizations require medication carts to be locked when not in use.

Careful handling and close observation prevent accidental or deliberate disarrangement of medications.

Check agency policy, which may allow for administration within a period of 30 minutes before or 30 minutes after designated time.

Identifying the patient ensures the right patient receives the medications and helps prevent errors.

This is the most reliable method. Replace the identification band if it is missing or inaccurate in any way.

This requires a response from the patient, but illness and strange surroundings often cause patients to be confused.

This is another way to double-check identity. Do not use the name on the door or over the bed, because these may be inaccurate.

This provides patient privacy.

Assessment is a prerequisite to administration of medications. Explanation provides rationale, increases knowledge, and reduces anxiety.

(continued)

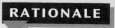

ACTION

17. Scan the patient's bar code on the identification band, if required.

18. Perform hand hygiene and put on clean gloves.

19. Select an appropriate administration site.

20. Assist the patient to the appropriate position for the site chosen. See Table 3. Drape as needed to expose only area of site to be used.

21. **Identify the appropriate landmarks for the site chosen.**

22. Clean the area around the injection site with an antimicrobial swab. Use a firm, circular motion while moving outward from the injection site. Allow area to dry.

23. Remove the needle cap by pulling it straight off. Hold the syringe in your dominant hand between the thumb and forefinger.

24. Displace the skin in a Z-track manner by pulling the skin down or to one side about 1″ (2.5 cm) with your nondominant hand and hold the skin and tissue in this position (Figure 2). (See the accompanying Skill Variation for information on administering an intramuscular injection without using the Z-track technique.)

RATIONALE

Provides additional check to ensure that the medication is given to the right patient.

Hand hygiene prevents the spread of microorganisms. Gloves help prevent exposure to contaminants.

Selecting the appropriate site prevents injury.

Good visualization is necessary to establish the correct location of the site and avoid damage to tissues.

Pathogens on the skin can be forced into the tissues by the needle. Moving from the center outward prevents contamination of the site. Allowing skin to dry prevents introducing alcohol into the tissue, which can be irritating and uncomfortable.

This technique lessens the risk of an accidental needlestick and also prevents inadvertently unscrewing the needle from the barrel of the syringe.

This ensures medication does not leak back along the needle track and into the subcutaneous tissue.

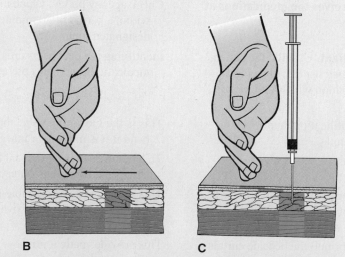

A   B   C   D

Figure 2. The Z-track or zigzag technique is recommended for intramuscular injections. (**A**) Normal skin and tissues. (**B**) Moving the skin to one side. (**C**) Needle is inserted at a 90-degree angle, and the nurse aspirates for blood. (**D**) Once the needle is withdrawn, displaced tissue is allowed to return to its normal position, preventing the solution from escaping from the muscle tissue.

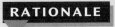

SKILL
7   **Administering an Intramuscular Injection** (continued)

ACTION

25. Quickly dart the needle into the tissue so that the needle is perpendicular to the patient's body (Figure 3). This should ensure that it is given using an angle of injection between 72 to 90 degrees.

26. As soon as the needle is in place, use your thumb and forefinger of your nondominant hand to hold the lower end of the syringe. Slide your dominant hand to the end of the plunger.

27. **Aspirate by slowly (for at least 5 seconds) pulling back on the plunger to determine whether the needle is in a blood vessel (Figure 4). Watch for a flash of pink or red in the syringe.**

RATIONALE

A quick injection is less painful. Inserting the needle at a 72-to-90-degree angle facilitates entry into muscle tissue.

Moving the syringe could cause damage to the tissues and inadvertent administration into incorrect area.

Discomfort and possibly a serious reaction may occur if a drug intended for intramuscular use is injected into a vein. Allowing slow aspiration facilitates backflow of blood even if needle is in a small, low-flow blood vessel.

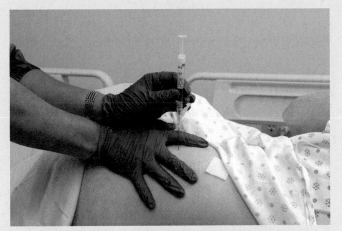

Figure 3. Darting the needle into the tissue.

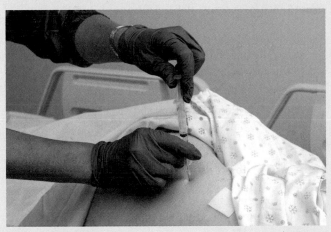

Figure 4. Aspirating.

28. If no blood is aspirated, inject the solution slowly (10 seconds per milliliter of medication).

29. Once the medication has been instilled, wait 10 seconds before withdrawing the needle.

30. Withdraw the needle smoothly and steadily at the same angle at which it was inserted, supporting tissue around the injection site with your nondominant hand.

31. **Apply gentle pressure at the site with a dry gauze (Figure 5).**

Rapid injection of the solution creates pressure in the tissues, resulting in discomfort.

Allows medication to begin to diffuse into the surrounding muscle tissue (Nicoll & Hesby, 2002)

Slow withdrawal of the needle pulls the tissues and causes discomfort. Applying counter traction around the injection site helps to prevent pulling on the tissue as the needle is withdrawn. Removing the needle at the same angle at which it was inserted minimizes tissue damage and discomfort for the patient.

Light pressure causes less trauma and irritation to the tissues. Massaging can force medication into subcutaneous tissues.

(continued)

Administering an Intramuscular Injection (continued)

ACTION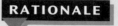

RATIONALE

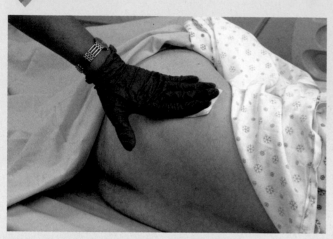

Figure 5. Applying pressure at the injection site.

32. Do not recap the used needle. Engage the safety shield or needle guard, if present. Discard the needle and syringe in the appropriate receptacle.

Proper disposal of the needle prevents injury.

33. Assist the patient to a position of comfort.

This provides for the well-being of the patient.

34. Remove gloves and dispose of them properly. Perform hand hygiene.

Hand hygiene deters the spread of microorganisms.

35. Evaluate patient's response to medication within an appropriate time frame. Assess site, if possible, within 2 to 4 hours after administration.

Evaluates effectiveness of drug and provides early detection of adverse effect. Adverse reaction to medication given by the parenteral route is a possibility. Visualization of the site also allows for assessment of any untoward effects.

EVALUATION

The expected outcomes are met when the patient receives the medication via the intramuscular route; the patient's anxiety is decreased; the patient does not experience adverse effects or injury; and the patient understands and complies with the medication regimen.

Documentation

Guidelines

Record each medication given on the MAR or record using the required format, including date, time and the site of administration, immediately after administration. If using a bar-code system, medication administration is automatically recorded when scanned. PRN medications require documentation of the reason for administration. Prompt recording avoids the possibility of accidentally repeating the administration of the drug. If the drug was refused or omitted, record this in the appropriate area on the medication record and notify the physician. This verifies the reason medication was omitted and ensures that the physician is aware of the patient's condition.

Unexpected Situations and Associated Interventions

• *Nurse sticks self with needle before injection:* Discard needle and syringe appropriately. Follow agency policy regarding needlestick injury. Prepare new syringe with medication and administer to patient. Complete appropriate paperwork and follow agency's policy regarding accidental needlesticks.

Administering an Intramuscular Injection *(continued)*

- *Nurse sticks self with needle after injection:* Discard needle and syringe appropriately. Follow agency policy regarding needlestick injury. Complete appropriate paperwork and follow agency's policy regarding accidental needlesticks.
- *During injection, patient pulls away from needle before medication is delivered fully:* Remove and appropriately discard needle. Attach a new needle to syringe and administer remaining medication at a different site. Document events and interventions according to facility policy.
- *While injecting needle into patient, nurse hits patient's bone:* Withdraw and discard the needle. Apply new needle to syringe and administer in alternate site. Document incident in patient's notes. Notify physician. Complete appropriate paperwork related to adverse events according to facility policy.

Special Considerations

General Considerations

Ongoing assessment is an important part of nursing care to evaluate patient response to administered medications and early detection of adverse effects. If an adverse effect is suspected, withhold further medication doses and notify the patient's primary healthcare provider. Additional intervention is based on type of reaction and patient assessment.

Infant and Child Considerations

- The vastus lateralis is the preferred site for infants.

Older Adult Considerations

- Muscle mass atrophies as a person ages. Take care to evaluate the patient's muscle mass and body composition. Use appropriate needle length and gauge for patient's body composition. Choose appropriate site based on the patient's body composition.

Home Care Considerations

- Encourage patients to consult the policies of their local government regarding contaminated and sharps waste disposal. Needles and syringes should be disposed of in a hard, plastic container. Liquid detergent or liquid fabric softener containers are good choices. Glass containers should not be used.

SKILL VARIATION Administering an Intramuscular Injection Without Using the Z-Track Technique

If the Z-Track technique is not used, the skin is stretched flat between two fingers and held taut for needle insertion. To administer the injection:

- Perform hand hygiene and put on clean gloves.
- Select an appropriate administration site.
- Assist the patient to the appropriate position for the site chosen. Drape as needed to expose only area of site to be used.
- Identify the appropriate landmarks for the site chosen with your nondominant hand.
- Clean the area around the injection site with an antimicrobial swab. Use a firm, circular motion while moving outward from the injection site. Allow area to dry.
- Remove the needle cap by pulling it straight off. Hold the syringe in your dominant hand between the thumb and forefinger.
- Stretch the skin flat between two fingers and hold taut for needle insertion.
- Quickly dart the needle into the tissue so that the needle is perpendicular to the patient's body. This should ensure that it is given using an angle of injection between 72 to 90 degrees.

- As soon as the needle is in place, use your thumb and forefinger of your nondominant hand to hold the lower end of the syringe. Slide your dominant hand to the end of the plunger.
- Aspirate by slowly (for at least 5 seconds) pulling back on the plunger to determine whether the needle is in a blood vessel. Watch for a flash of pink or red in the syringe.
- If no blood is aspirated, inject the solution slowly (10 seconds per mL of medication)
- Withdraw the needle smoothly and steadily at the same angle at which it was inserted, supporting tissue around the injection site with your nondominant hand.
- Apply gentle pressure at the site with a dry gauze.
- Do not recap the used needle. Engage the safety shield or needle guard, if present. Discard the needle and syringe in the appropriate receptacle.
- Assist the patient to a position of comfort.
- Remove gloves and dispose of them properly. Perform hand hygiene.
- Evaluate patient's response to medication within an appropriate time frame. Assess site, if possible, within 2 to 4 hours after administration.

Administering Continuous Subcutaneous Infusion: Applying an Insulin Pump

Some medications, such as insulin, may be administered continuously via the subcutaneous route. Continuous subcutaneous insulin infusion (CSII or insulin pump) allows for multiple preset rates of insulin delivery. This system uses a small computerized reservoir that delivers insulin via tubing through a needle inserted into the subcutaneous tissue. The pump is programmed to deliver multiple preset rates of insulin delivery. The settings can be adjusted for exercise and illness, and bolus dose delivery can be timed in relation to meals. Change sites every two to three days to prevent tissue damage or absorption problems (Olohan & Zappitelli, 2003). Advantages of continuous subcutaneous medication infusion include the longer rate of absorption via the subcutaneous route and convenience for the patient.

Equipment

- Insulin pump
- Pump syringe
- Vial of insulin as ordered
- Sterile infusion set
- Insertion (triggering) device
- Needle (24 or 22 gauge, or blunt-ended needle)
- Antimicrobial swabs
- Sterile nonocclusive dressing
- Medication Administration Record (MAR) or Computer-generated MAR (CMAR)
- Clean gloves

ASSESSMENT

Assess the patient for any allergies. Check expiration date before administering medication. Assess the appropriateness of the drug for the patient. Review assessment and laboratory data that may influence drug administration. Verify patient name, dose, route, and time of administration. Assess skin in the area where the pump is to be applied. The pump should not be placed on skin that is irritated or broken down. Assess the patient's knowledge of the medication. If the patient has a knowledge deficit about the medication, this may be the appropriate time to begin education about the medication. If the medication may affect the patient's vital signs, assess them before administration. If the medication is for pain relief, assess the patient's pain level before and after administration. Assess the patient's blood glucose level as appropriate or as ordered.

NURSING DIAGNOSIS

Determine related factors for the nursing diagnoses based on the patient's current status. Appropriate nursing diagnoses may include:

- Deficient Knowledge
- Risk for Allergy Response
- Risk for Impaired Skin Integrity
- Acute Pain
- Risk for Infection

OUTCOME IDENTIFICATION AND PLANNING

The expected outcome is that the device is applied successfully and medication is administered. Other outcomes that may be appropriate include the following: patient understands the rationale for the pump use and mechanism of action; patient experiences no allergy response; patient's skin remains intact; pump is applied using aseptic technique; and patient does not experience adverse effect.

SKILL 8

Administering Continuous Subcutaneous Infusion: Applying an Insulin Pump *(continued)*

IMPLEMENTATION

ACTION	**RATIONALE**
1. Gather equipment. Check each medication order against the original physician's order according to agency policy. Clarify any inconsistencies. Check the patient's chart for allergies.	This comparison helps to identify errors that may have occurred when orders were transcribed. The physician's order is the legal record of medication orders for each agency.
2. Know the actions, special nursing considerations, safe dose ranges, purpose of administration, and adverse effects of the medications to be administered. Consider the appropriateness of the medication for this patient.	This knowledge aids the nurse in evaluating the therapeutic effect of the medication in relation to the patient's disorder and can also be used to educate the patient about the medication.
3. Perform hand hygiene.	Hand hygiene prevents the spread of microorganisms.
4. Move the medication cart to the outside of the patient's room or prepare for administration in the medication area.	Organization facilitates error-free administration and saves time.
5. Unlock the medication cart or drawer. Enter pass code and scan employee identification, if required.	Locking of the cart or drawer safeguards each patient's medication supply. Hospital accrediting organizations require medication carts to be locked when not in use. Entering pass code and scanning ID allows only authorized users into the system and identifies user for documentation by the computer.
6. **Prepare medications for one patient at a time.**	This prevents errors in medication administration.
7. Read the MAR and select the proper medication from the patient's medication drawer or unit stock.	This is the first check of the label.
8. Compare the label with the MAR. Check expiration dates and perform calculations, if necessary. Scan the bar code on the package, if required.	This is the second check of the label. Verify calculations with another nurse to ensure safety, if necessary.
9. Attach blunt-ended needle or small-gauge needle to syringe. Follow Skill 3 to remove insulin from vial. Remove enough insulin to last patient 2 to 3 days, plus 30 units for priming tubing.	Patient will wear pump for up to 3 days without changing syringe or tubing.
10. **When all medications for one patient have been prepared, recheck the label with the MAR before taking them to the patient.**	This is a *third* check to ensure accuracy and to prevent errors.
11. Lock the medication cart before leaving it.	Locking the cart or drawer safeguards the patient's medication supply. Hospital accrediting organizations require medication carts to be locked when not in use.
12. Transport medications to the patient's bedside carefully, and keep the medications in sight at all times.	Careful handling and close observation prevent accidental or deliberate disarrangement of medications.
13. **Ensure that the patient receives the medications at the correct time.**	Check agency policy, which may allow for administration within a period of 30 minutes before or 30 minutes after designated time.

(continued)

ACTION

RATIONALE

14. **Identify the patient.** Usually, the patient should be identified using two methods. Compare information with the MAR or CMAR.

Identifying the patient ensures the right patient receives the medications and helps prevent errors.

a. Check the name and identification number on the patient's identification band.

This is the most reliable method. Replace the identification band if it is missing or inaccurate in any way.

b. Ask the patient to state his or her name.

This requires a response from the patient, but illness and strange surroundings often cause patients to be confused.

c. If the patient cannot identify him or herself, verify the patient's identification with a staff member who knows the patient.

This is another way to double-check identity. Do not use the name on the door or over the bed, because these may be inaccurate.

15. Close the door to the room or pull the bedside curtain.

This provides patient privacy.

16. Complete necessary assessments before administering medications. Check allergy bracelet or ask patient about allergies. Explain the purpose and action of the medication to the patient.

Assessment is a prerequisite to administration of medications. Explanation provides rationale, increases knowledge, and reduces anxiety.

17. Scan the patient's bar code on the identification band, if required.

Provides additional check to ensure that the medication is given to the right patient.

18. Perform hand hygiene.

Hand hygiene prevents the spread of microorganisms.

19. Attach sterile tubing to syringe. Prime the tubing by pushing the plunger of syringe until insulin is coming from introducer needle (Figure 1). **Check for any bubbles in tubing.**

Removing all air from tubing ensures that patient receives the correct dose of insulin.

20. Program pump according to manufacturer's recommendations following physician's orders. Open pump and place syringe in compartment according to manufacturer's directions (Figure 2). Close pump.

Syringe must be placed in pump correctly for delivery of insulin.

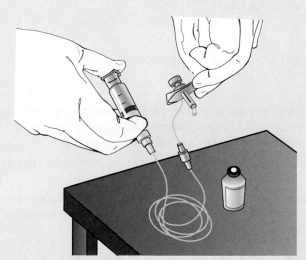

Figure 1. Priming insulin pump tubing.

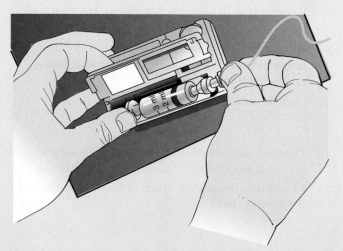

Figure 2. Placing syringe in compartment according to manufacturer's directions.

Administering Continuous Subcutaneous Infusion: Applying an Insulin Pump *(continued)*

ACTION	RATIONALE
21. Activate delivery device. Place needle between prongs of insertion device with sharp edge facing out. Push insertion set down until click is heard.	To ensure correct placement of insulin pump needle, insertion device must be used.
22. Put on clean gloves.	Gloves help prevent exposure to contaminants.
23. Select an appropriate administration site.	Appropriate site prevents injury.
24. Assist the patient to the appropriate position for the site chosen. Drape as needed to expose only area of site to be used.	Maintains privacy and warmth.
25. Identify the appropriate landmarks for the site chosen.	Good visualization is necessary to establish the correct location of the site and avoid damage to tissues.
26. Clean area around injection site with antimicrobial swab. Use a firm, circular motion while moving outward from insertion site (Figure 3). Allow antiseptic to dry.	Pathogens on the skin can be forced into the tissues by the needle. Moving from the center outward prevents contamination of the site. Allowing skin to dry prevents introducing alcohol into the tissue, which can be irritating and uncomfortable.
27. Remove paper from adhesive backing. Remove needle guard. Pinch skin at insertion site, press insertion device on site, and press release button to insert needle (Figure 4). Remove triggering device.	To ensure delivery of insulin into subcutaneous tissue, a skin fold is made with a pinch *before* insertion of the medication.

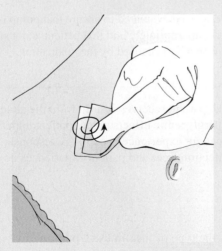

Figure 3. Cleaning area before insertion.

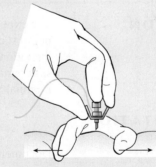

Figure 4. Inserting needle and delivery device.

28. **While holding needle hub, turn it a quarter-turn and remove needle (Figure 5).** Do not recap the used needle. Engage the safety shield or needle guard, if present.	The actual metal needle is removed and a plastic stylet is left in place to deliver the medication. If needle hub is not rotated, the stylet may be removed as well. Needle guards prevent injury.
29. Apply sterile occlusive dressing over insertion site (Figure 6). Attach the pump to patient's clothing.	Dressing prevents contamination of site. Pump can be dislodged easily if not attached securely to patient.

(continued)

Administering Continuous Subcutaneous Infusion: Applying an Insulin Pump *(continued)*

ACTION

RATIONALE

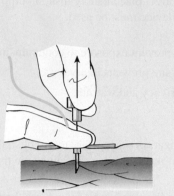

Figure 5. Removing needle from delivery device.

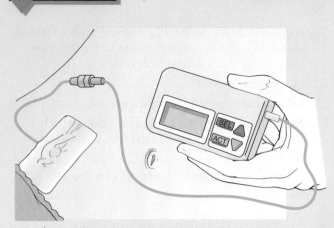

Figure 6. MiniMed insulin pump attached.

30. Discard the needle and syringe in the appropriate receptacle.

Proper disposal of the needle prevents injury.

31. Assist the patient to a position of comfort.

This provides for the well-being of the patient.

32. Remove gloves and dispose of them properly. Perform hand hygiene.

Hand hygiene deters the spread of microorganisms.

33. Evaluate patient's response to medication within appropriate time frame. Monitor the patient's blood glucose levels as appropriate or as ordered.

Patient needs to be evaluated to ensure that pump is delivering drug appropriately and that patient is not suffering any adverse affects caused by the medication.

EVALUATION

The expected outcomes are met when the patient receives insulin from the attached pump successfully without hypo- or hyperglycemic effects noted; patient understands the rationale for the pump attachment; patient experiences no allergy response; patient's skin remained intact; patient remains infection free; and patient experiences no or minimal pain.

DOCUMENTATION

Guidelines

Document the application of the pump, the type of insulin used, pump settings, insertion site, and any teaching done with patient on the MAR or record using the required format, including date, time and the site of administration, immediately after administration. If using a bar-code system, medication administration is automatically recorded when scanned. PRN medications require documentation of the reason for administration. Prompt recording avoids the possibility of accidentally repeating the administration of the drug. If the drug was refused or omitted, record this in the appropriate area on the medication record and notify the physician. This verifies the reason medication was omitted and ensures that the physician is aware of the patient's condition.

Administering Continuous Subcutaneous Infusion: Applying an Insulin Pump *(continued)*

Sample Documentation

9/22/08 1000 Insulin pump inserted by patient on LUQ of abdomen with minimal assistance. Pump filled with 300 units (3 mL) of lispro insulin. Rate set at 1 unit per hour. Patient verbalizes desire to apply pump without assistance when site next changed.—B. Clapp, RN

Unexpected Situations and Associated Interventions

- *After pump is attached to patient, a large amount of air is noted in tubing:* Remove pump from patient. Obtain new sterile tubing with insertion needle. Prime tubing and reinsert.
- *Patient must rotate site more frequently than every 2 to 3 days due to insulin usage:* Check manufacturer's recommendations. Most pumps are initially set in a smaller mode but can be changed for a large amount of insulin delivery.
- *Patient is refusing to rotate site at least every 3 days:* Inform patient that absorption of medication decreases after 3 days, which may increase his or her need for insulin. Rotating sites prevents this decrease in absorption from developing.
- *Nurse notes that insertion site is now erythematous:* Remove the stylet, obtain a new pump setup, and insert at a different site at least 1″ from old site.
- *Occlusive dressing will not stick due to perspiration:* Apply deodorant around insertion site but not over insertion site. Alternately, apply skin barrier around insertion site but not over insertion site.

Special Considerations

General Considerations

- Assess infusion site areas routinely for inflammation, allergic reactions, infection, and lipodystrophy.
- Good hygiene and frequent catheter site changes reduce risk of site complications. Change catheter site every 2 to 3 days.
- Contact dermatitis is sometimes a problem at the catheter site area. The physician or healthcare provider may order topical antibiotics, aloe, vitamin E, or corticosteroids to treat a contact dermatitis.
- Insulin self-administered by the patient through the insulin pump should be communicated to the nurse at the time of administration. This allows for accurate documentation of insulin requirements.
- Ongoing assessment is an important part of nursing care to evaluate patient response to administered medications and early detection of adverse effects. If an adverse effect is suspected, withhold further medication doses and notify the patient's primary healthcare provider. Additional intervention is based on type of reaction and patient assessment.

Home Care Considerations

- Encourage patients to consult the policies of their local government regarding contaminated and sharps waste disposal. Needles and other sharps should be disposed of in a hard, plastic container. Liquid detergent or liquid fabric softener containers are good choices. Glass containers should not be used.

Adding Medications to an Intravenous (IV) Solution Container

Medications may be added to the patient's infusion solution. The pharmacist commonly adds the prescribed drug to a large volume of IV solution, but sometimes the drug is added in the nursing unit, in which case sterile technique must be maintained.

When medication is administered by continuous infusion, the patient receives it slowly, over a long period. If the patient needs the medication quickly, this route/method should not be used. Consider also that if for some reason all of the solution cannot be infused, the patient will not receive the prescribed amount of the medication. Check a patient receiving medication by a continuous IV infusion for possible adverse effects at least every hour.

Equipment

- Prescribed medication
- Syringe with a 19- to 21-gauge needle, blunt needle, or needleless device (follow agency policy)
- IV fluid container (bag or bottle)
- Antimicrobial swab
- Label to be attached to the IV fluid container
- Medication Administration Record (MAR) or Computer-generated MAR (CMAR)

ASSESSMENT

Assess the patient for any allergies. Check expiration date before administering medication. Assess the appropriateness of the drug for the patient. Assess the compatibility of the ordered medication and the IV fluid. Review assessment and laboratory data that may influence drug administration. Verify patient name, dose, route, and time of administration. Assess the patient's knowledge of the medication. If the patient has a knowledge deficit about the medication, this may be the appropriate time to begin education about the medication. If the medication may affect the patient's vital signs, assess them before administration. Assess the IV insertion site, noting any swelling, coolness, leakage of fluid at site, redness, or pain.

NURSING DIAGNOSIS

Determine related factors for the nursing diagnoses based on the patient's current status. Appropriate nursing diagnoses may include:

- Risk for Injury
- Risk for Allergy Response
- Risk for Infection
- Deficient Knowledge
- Anxiety

OUTCOME IDENTIFICATION AND PLANNING

The expected outcome is that the medication is added to an adequate amount of compatible solution and mixed appropriately. Other outcomes that may be appropriate include the following: medication is delivered to the patient in a safe manner and at the appropriate infusion rate; patient experiences no allergy response; patient remains infection free; and the patient understands and complies with the medication regimen.

IMPLEMENTATION

ACTION

1. Gather equipment. Check medication order against the original physician's order according to agency policy. Clarify any inconsistencies. Check the patient's chart for allergies. Verify the compatibility of the medication and IV fluid. Calculate the infusion rate.

RATIONALE

This comparison helps to identify errors that may have occurred when orders were transcribed. The physician's order is the legal record of medication orders for each agency. Compatibility of medication and solution prevents complications. Delivers the correct dose of medication as prescribed.

Adding Medications to an Intravenous (IV) Solution Container *(continued)*

ACTION	**RATIONALE**
2. Know the actions, special nursing considerations, safe dose ranges, purpose of administration, and adverse effects of the medications to be administered. Consider the appropriateness of the medication for this patient.	This knowledge aids the nurse in evaluating the therapeutic effect of the medication in relation to the patient's disorder and can also be used to educate the patient about the medication.
3. Perform hand hygiene.	Hand hygiene prevents the spread of microorganisms.
4. Move the medication cart to the outside of the patient's room or prepare for administration in the medication area.	Organization facilitates error-free administration and saves time.
5. Unlock the medication cart or drawer. Enter pass code and scan employee identification, if required.	Locking of the cart or drawer safeguards each patient's medication supply. Hospital accrediting organizations require medication carts to be locked when not in use. Entering pass code and scanning ID allows only authorized users into the system and identifies user for documentation by the computer.
6. **Prepare medication for one patient at a time.**	This prevents errors in medication administration.
7. Read the MAR and select the proper medication from the patient's medication drawer or unit stock.	This is the first check of the label.
8. Compare the label with the MAR. Check expiration dates and perform calculations, if necessary. Scan the bar code on the package, if required.	This is the second check of the label. Verify calculations with another nurse to ensure safety, if necessary.
9. If necessary, withdraw medication from an ampule or vial as described in Skills 2 and 3.	
10. **Recheck the label with the MAR before taking it to the patient.**	This is a *third* check to ensure accuracy and to prevent errors.
11. Lock the medication cart before leaving it.	Locking the cart or drawer safeguards the patient's medication supply. Hospital accrediting organizations require medication carts to be locked when not in use.
12. Transport medications and equipment to the patient's bedside carefully, and keep the medications in sight at all times.	Careful handling and close observation prevent accidental or deliberate disarrangement of medications. Having equipment available saves time and facilitates performance of the task.
13. Perform hand hygiene.	Hand hygiene deters the spread of microorganisms.
14. **Identify the patient.** Usually, the patient should be identified using two methods. Compare information with the MAR or CMAR.	Identifying the patient ensures the right patient receives the medications and helps prevent errors.
a. Check the name and identification number on the patient's identification band.	This is the most reliable method. Replace the identification band if it is missing or inaccurate in any way.

(continued)

Adding Medications to an Intravenous (IV) Solution Container *(continued)*

ACTION	**RATIONALE**

b. Ask the patient to state his or her name.

This requires a response from the patient, but illness and strange surroundings often cause patients to be confused.

c. If the patient cannot identify him or herself, verify the patient's identification with a staff member who knows the patient for the second source.

This is another way to double-check identity. Do not use the name on the door or over the bed, because these may be inaccurate.

15. Close the door to the room or pull the bedside curtain.

This provides patient privacy.

16. Complete necessary assessments before administering medications. Check allergy bracelet or ask patient about allergies. Explain the purpose and action of the medication to the patient.

Assessment is a prerequisite to administration of medications. Explanation provides rationale, increases knowledge, and reduces anxiety.

17. Scan the patient's bar code on the identification band, if required.

Provides additional check to ensure that the medication is given to the right patient.

18. **Check that the volume in the current IV infusion is adequate.** (See the accompanying Skill Variation for information on adding medication to a new IV container.)

The volume should be sufficient to dilute the drug.

19. Close the clamp between the solution container and roller clamp on the infusion tubing (Figure 1) and pause the IV pump, if appropriate.

This prevents back-flow directly to the patient of improperly diluted medication.

20. Clean the medication port with an antimicrobial swab (Figure 2).

This deters entry of microorganisms when the port is punctured.

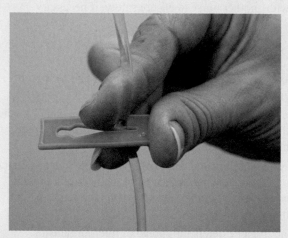
Figure 1. Closing the clamp on the infusion tubing.

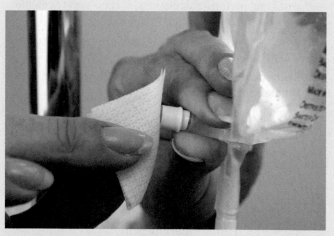
Figure 2. Cleaning the medication port.

21. Steady the container and uncap the needle or needleless device. Insert it into the port (Figure 3). Inject the medication. Withdraw the needle or needleless device. Do not recap the used needle. Engage the safety shield or needle guard, if present.

This ensures that the needle or needleless device enters the container and medication can be dispersed into the solution. Use of safety shield or needle guard prevents accidental injury.

22. Remove the container from the IV pole and gently rotate the container to mix the medication and solution (Figure 4).

This mixes the medication with the solution.

Adding Medications to an Intravenous (IV) Solution Container *(continued)*

ACTION

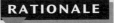**RATIONALE**

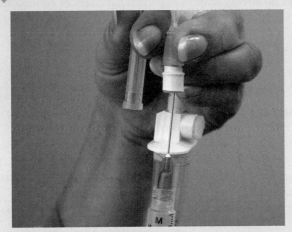

Figure 3. Inserting the needle into the port.

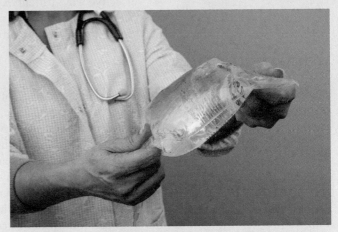

Figure 4. Rotating the container to mix the medication and solution.

23. Rehang the container on the pole. **Attach the label to the container so that the dose of medication that has been added is apparent (Figure 5).**

24. Open the clamp, and readjust the flow rate (Figure 6) or check the pump settings for correct infusion rate and restart pump.

This confirms that the prescribed dose of medication has been added to the IV solution.

Ensures the infusion of the IV with the medication at the prescribed rate.

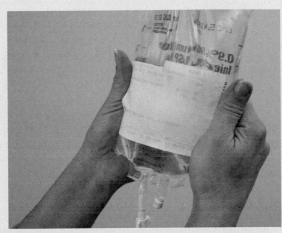

Figure 5. Labeling container to show medication addition.

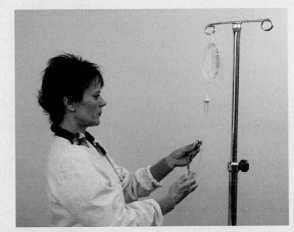

Figure 6. Readjusting flow rate.

25. Discard the needle and syringe in the appropriate receptacle.

26. Perform hand hygiene.

27. Evaluate the patient's response to medication within the appropriate time frame.

Proper disposal of the needle prevents injury.

This prevents spread of microorganisms.

Patients require careful observation because medications given by the IV route may have a rapid effect.

(continued)

SKILL 9

Adding Medications to an Intravenous (IV) Solution Container *(continued)*

EVALUATION

The expected outcomes are met when the medication is added to an adequate amount of IV solution and mixed appropriately; patient receives the medication in a safe and effective way; patient experiences no allergy response; patient experiences no infection; patient understands reasons for procedure; and patient experiences decreased anxiety regarding medication infusion.

DOCUMENTATION

Guidelines

Document the addition of the medication to the IV solution immediately after administration, including date, time, dose, route of administration, site of administration, and rate of administration on the MAR or record using the required format. If using a bar-code system, medication administration is automatically recorded when scanned. PRN medications require documentation of the reason for administration. Prompt recording avoids the possibility of accidentally repeating the administration of the drug. If the drug was refused or omitted, record this in the appropriate area on the medication record and notify the physician. This verifies the reason medication was omitted and ensures that the physician is aware of the patient's condition.

Unexpected Situations and Associated Interventions

- *There is not enough IV solution in container:* Obtain new IV fluid container from medication station and add medication. Remove current IV bag and replace with newly admixed IV fluid. (Some institutions would prefer that the pharmacy mix any new bags so that the process may be done in a sterile environment.)
- *Nurse realizes that wrong medication or wrong amount of medication was added to the IV bag:* Immediately stop infusion. Assess patient for any distress and notify physician. Follow agency policy for medication error. Remove bag of IV fluids and replace with IV containing ordered medication.
- *Nurse sticks self with needle while trying to inject medication into port:* Discard syringe and needle. Prepare new syringe with medication.
- *Needle goes through side of medication injection port:* Discard syringe, needle, and current bag of IV solution. Replace with newly mixed IV fluid. (Some institutions would prefer pharmacy mix any new bags so that the process may be done in a sterile environment.)

Special Considerations

General Considerations

- Ongoing assessment is an important part of nursing care to evaluate patient response to administered medications and early detection of adverse effects. If an adverse effect is suspected, withhold further medication doses and notify the patient's primary healthcare provider. Additional intervention is based on type of reaction and patient assessment.

Adding Medications to an Intravenous (IV) Solution Container *(continued)*

SKILL VARIATION Adding Medication to a New Intravenous Container

- Check medication order against the original physician's order according to agency policy. Clarify any inconsistencies. Check the patient's chart for allergies. Verify the compatibility of the medication and IV fluid. Calculate the infusion rate.
- Know the actions, special nursing considerations, safe dose ranges, purpose of administration, and adverse effects of the medications to be administered. Consider the appropriateness of the medication for this patient.
- Perform hand hygiene.
- Move the medication cart to the outside of the patient's room or prepare for administration in the medication area.
- Unlock the medication cart or drawer. Enter pass code and scan employee identification, if required.
- Read the MAR and select the proper medication from the patient's medication drawer or unit stock.
- Compare the label with the MAR. Check expiration dates and perform calculations, if necessary. Scan the bar code on the package, if required.
- If necessary, withdraw medication from an ampule or vial as described in Skills 2 and 3.
- Recheck the label with the MAR before taking it to the patient.
- Lock the medication cart before leaving it.
- Transport medications and equipment to the patient's bedside carefully, and keep the medications in sight at all times.
- Perform hand hygiene.

- Identify the patient. Usually, the patient should be identified using two methods.
- Close the door to the room or pull the bedside curtain.
- Complete necessary assessments before administering medications. Check allergy bracelet or ask patient about allergies. Explain the purpose and action of the medication to the patient.
- Scan the patient's bar code on the identification band, if required.
- Carefully remove any protective cover and locate the injection port. Clean with an antimicrobial swab.
- Uncap the needle or needleless device and insert into the port. Inject the medication.
- Gently rotate the IV solution in the bag or bottle.
- Attach the label to the container so that the dose of medication that has been added is apparent.
- Do not recap the used needle. Engage the safety shield or needle guard, if present. Discard the needle and syringe in the appropriate receptacle.
- Perform hand hygiene.
- Prepare the IV infusion for administration according to facility policy.
- Evaluate the patient's response to medication within the appropriate time frame.

SKILL 10 Administering Medications by Intravenous Bolus or Push Through an Intravenous Infusion

A medication can be administered as an IV bolus or push. This involves a single injection of a concentrated solution directly into an IV line. Drugs given by IV push are used for intermittent dosing or to treat emergencies. The drug is administered very slowly over at least one minute. Exact administration times should be confirmed by consulting a pharmacist or drug reference.

Equipment

- Antimicrobial swab
- Watch with second hand, or stopwatch
- Clean gloves
- Prescribed medication
- Syringe with a needleless device or 23- to 25-gauge, 1″ needle (follow agency policy)
- Medication Administration Record (MAR) or Computer-generated MAR (CMAR)

ASSESSMENT

Assess the patient for any allergies. Check expiration date before administering medication. Assess the appropriateness of the drug for the patient. Assess the compatibility of the ordered medication and the IV fluid. Review assessment and laboratory data that may influence drug administration. Verify the patient's name, dose, route, and time of adminis-

(continued)

tration. Assess patient's IV site, noting any swelling, coolness, leakage of fluid from IV site, or pain. Assess the patient's knowledge of the medication. If the patient has a knowledge deficit about the medication, this may be the appropriate time to begin education about the medication. If the medication may affect the patient's vital signs, assess them before administration.

NURSING DIAGNOSIS

Determine related factors for the nursing diagnoses based on the patient's current status. Appropriate nursing diagnoses may include:

- Acute Pain
- Risk for Allergy Response
- Deficient Knowledge
- Risk for Infection
- Anxiety
- Risk for Injury

OUTCOME IDENTIFICATION AND PLANNING

The expected outcome to achieve is that the medication is given safely. Other outcomes that may be appropriate include the following: patient experiences no adverse effect; patient experiences no allergy response; patient is knowledgeable about medication being added by bolus IV; patient remains infection free; and patient has no, or decreased, anxiety.

IMPLEMENTATION

ACTION

RATIONALE

1. Gather equipment. Check medication order against the original physician's order according to agency policy. Clarify any inconsistencies. Check the patient's chart for allergies. Verify the compatibility of the medication and IV fluid. Check a drug resource to clarify whether medication needs to be diluted before administration. Check the infusion rate.

This comparison helps to identify errors that may have occurred when orders were transcribed. The physician's order is the legal record of medication orders for each agency. Compatibility of medication and solution prevents complications. Delivers the correct dose of medication as prescribed.

2. Know the actions, special nursing considerations, safe dose ranges, purpose of administration, and adverse effects of the medications to be administered. Consider the appropriateness of the medication for this patient.

This knowledge aids the nurse in evaluating the therapeutic effect of the medication in relation to the patient's disorder and can also be used to educate the patient about the medication.

3. Perform hand hygiene.

Hand hygiene prevents the spread of microorganisms.

4. Move the medication cart to the outside of the patient's room or prepare for administration in the medication area.

Organization facilitates error-free administration and saves time.

5. Unlock the medication cart or drawer. Enter pass code and scan employee identification, if required.

Locking of the cart or drawer safeguards each patient's medication supply. Hospital accrediting organizations require medication carts to be locked when not in use. Entering pass code and scanning ID allows only authorized users into the system and identifies user for documentation by the computer.

SKILL 10

Administering Medications by Intravenous Bolus or Push Through an Intravenous Infusion *(continued)*

ACTION	RATIONALE
6. **Prepare medication for one patient at a time.**	This prevents errors in medication administration.
7. Read the MAR and select the proper medication from the patient's medication drawer or unit stock.	This is the first check of the label.
8. Compare the label with the MAR. Check expiration dates and perform calculations, if necessary. Scan the bar code on the package, if required.	This is the second check of the label. Verify calculations with another nurse to ensure safety, if necessary.
9. If necessary, withdraw medication from an ampule or vial as described in Skills 2 and 3.	
10. **Recheck the label with the MAR before taking it to the patient.**	This is a *third* check to ensure accuracy and to prevent errors.
11. Lock the medication cart before leaving it.	Locking the cart or drawer safeguards the patient's medication supply. Hospital accrediting organizations require medication carts to be locked when not in use.
12. Transport medications and equipment to the patient's bedside carefully, and keep the medications in sight at all times.	Careful handling and close observation prevent accidental or deliberate disarrangement of medications. Having equipment available saves time and facilitates performance of the task.
13. Perform hand hygiene.	Hand hygiene deters the spread of microorganisms.
14. **Identify the patient.** Usually, the patient should be identified using two methods. Compare information with the MAR or CMAR.	Identifying the patient ensures the right patient receives the medications and helps prevent errors.
a. Check the name and identification number on the patient's identification band.	This is the most reliable method. Replace the identification band if it is missing or inaccurate in any way.
b. Ask the patient to state his or her name.	This requires a response from the patient, but illness and strange surroundings often cause patients to be confused.
c. If the patient cannot identify him or herself, verify the patient's identification with a staff member who knows the patient for the second source.	This is another way to double-check identity. Do not use the name on the door or over the bed, because these may be inaccurate.
15. Close the door to the room or pull the bedside curtain.	This provides patient privacy.
16. Complete necessary assessments before administering medications. Check allergy bracelet or ask patient about allergies. Explain the purpose and action of the medication to the patient.	Assessment is a prerequisite to administration of medications. Explanation provides rationale, increases knowledge, and reduces anxiety.
17. Scan the patient's bar code on the identification band, if required.	Provides additional check to ensure that the medication is given to the right patient.
18. **Assess IV site for presence of inflammation or infiltration.**	IV medication must be given directly into a vein for safe administration.
19. If IV infusion is being administered via an infusion pump, pause the pump.	Pausing prevents infusion of fluid during bolus administration and activation of pump occlusion alarms.
20. Put on clean gloves.	Gloves prevent contact with blood and body fluids.

(continued)

Administering Medications by Intravenous Bolus or Push Through an Intravenous Infusion *(continued)*

ACTION

21. Select injection port on tubing that is closest to venipuncture site. Clean port with antimicrobial swab (Figure 1).

22. Uncap syringe. Steady port with your nondominant hand while inserting syringe, needleless device, or needle into center of port (Figure 2).

RATIONALE

Using port closest to needle insertion site minimizes dilution of medication. Cleaning deters entry of microorganisms when port is punctured.

This supports injection port and lessens risk for accidentally dislodging IV or entering port incorrectly.

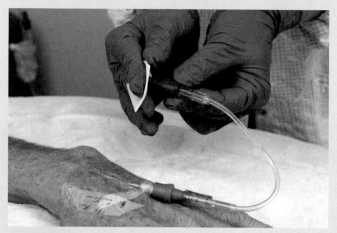

Figure 1. Cleaning injection port.

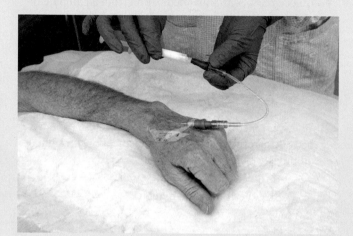

Figure 2. Inserting syringe into port.

23. Move your nondominant hand to section of IV tubing just above the injection port. Fold tubing between your fingers (Figure 3).

24. Pull back slightly on plunger just until blood appears in tubing.

25. **Inject medication at recommended rate** (see Special Considerations below) (Figure 4).

This temporarily stops flow of gravity IV infusion and prevents medication from backing up tubing.

This ensures injection of medication into the bloodstream.

This delivers correct amount of medication at proper interval according to manufacturer's directions.

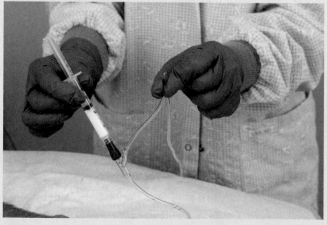

Figure 3. Folding tubing above port between fingers.

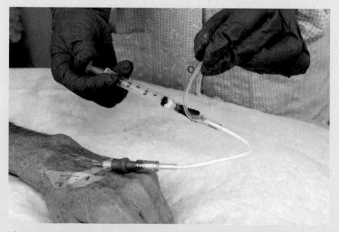

Figure 4. Injecting medication while interrupting IV flow.

ACTION	RATIONALE
26. Release the tubing. Remove the syringe. Do not recap the used needle. Engage the safety shield or needle guard, if present. Release the tubing and allow the IV fluid to flow. Discard the needle and syringe in the appropriate receptacle.	Proper disposal of the needle prevents injury.
27. Check IV fluid infusion rate. Restart infusion pump, if appropriate.	Injection of bolus may alter rate of fluid infusion, if infusing by gravity.
28. Remove gloves and perform hand hygiene.	Hand hygiene deters spread of microorganisms.
29. Evaluate patient's response to medication within appropriate time frame.	Patient requires careful observation because medications given by IV bolus injection may have a rapid effect.

EVALUATION

The expected outcomes are met when the medication is safely administered via IV bolus; the patient's anxiety is decreased; the patient does not experience adverse effects; and the patient understands and complies with the medication regimen.

DOCUMENTATION

Guidelines

Document the administration of the medication immediately after administration, including date, time, dose, route of administration, site of administration, and rate of administration on the MAR or record using the required format. If using a bar-code system, medication administration is automatically recorded when scanned. PRN medications require documentation of the reason for administration. Prompt recording avoids the possibility of accidentally repeating the administration of the drug. If the drug was refused or omitted, record this in the appropriate area on the medication record and notify the physician. This verifies the reason medication was omitted and ensures that the physician is aware of the patient's condition.

Unexpected Situations and Associated Interventions

- *Upon assessing IV site before administering medication, no blood return is aspirated:* If IV appears patent, without signs of infiltration, and IV fluid infuses without difficulty, proceed with administration. Observe closely for signs and symptoms of infiltration during and after administration.
- *Upon assessing patient's IV site before administering medication, nurse notes that IV has infiltrated:* Stop IV fluid and remove IV from extremity. Restart IV in a different location. Continue to monitor new IV site as medication is administered.
- *While administering medication, nurse notes a cloudy, white substance forming in IV tubing:* Stop IV from flowing and stop administering medication. Clamp IV at site nearest to patient. Change administration tubing and restart infusion. Check literature or consult pharmacist regarding compatibility of medication and IV fluid.
- *While nurse is administering medication, patient begins to complain of pain at IV site:* Stop medication. Assess IV site for any signs of infiltration or phlebitis. You may want to flush the IV with normal saline to check for patency. If the IV site appears within normal limits, resume medication administration at a slower rate.

(continued)

Administering Medications by Intravenous Bolus or Push Through an Intravenous Infusion *(continued)*

Special Considerations

General Considerations

- Agency policy may recommend the following variations when injecting a bolus IV medication:
  - Release folded tubing after each increment of the drug has been administered at prescribed rate to facilitate delivery of medication.
  - Use a syringe with 1 mL normal saline to flush tubing after an IV bolus is delivered to ensure that residual medication in tubing is not delivered too rapidly.
- Consider how fast IV fluid is flowing to determine whether a flush of normal saline is in order after administering medication. If IV fluid is flowing less than 50 mL per hour, it may take medication up to 30 minutes to reach patient. This depends on what type of tubing is being used in the agency.
- If the IV is a small gauge (22- to 24-gauge) placed in a small vein, a blood return may not occur even if IV is intact. Also, patient may complain of stinging and pain at site while medication is being administered due to irritation of vein. Placing a warm pack over vein or slowing the rate may relieve discomfort.
- If the medication and IV solution are incompatible, bolus may be given by flushing the tubing with normal saline before and after the medication bolus. Consult facility policy.
- Ongoing assessment is an important part of nursing care to evaluate patient response to administered medications and early detection of adverse effects. If an adverse effect is suspected, withhold further medication doses and notify the patient's primary healthcare provider. Additional intervention is based on type of reaction and patient assessment.

Administering a Piggyback Intermittent Intravenous Infusion of Medication

Watch & Learn

With intermittent IV infusion, the drug is mixed with a small amount of the IV solution, such as 50 to 100 mL, and administered over a short period at the prescribed interval (eg, every 4 hours). Medication may be administered by gravity infusion, which requires the nurse to calculate the infusion rate in drops per minute, or it may be administered using an IV infusion pump, which requires the nurse to program the infusion rate into the pump. 'Smart (computerized) pumps' are beginning to be used by many facilities for IV infusions, including intermittent infusions. 'Smart pumps' also requiring programming of infusion rates by the nurse, but, in addition, are able to identify dosing limits and practice guidelines to aid in safe administration. Needleless devices (recommended by the Centers for Disease Control and Prevention and the Occupational Safety and Health Administration) prevent needlesticks and provide access to the primary venous line. Either blunt-ended cannulas or recessed connection ports may be used to connect intermittent IV infusions.

The IV piggyback delivery system requires the intermittent or additive solution to be placed higher than the primary solution container. An extension hook provided by the manufacturer provides for easy lowering of the main IV container. The port on the primary IV line has a back-check valve that automatically stops the flow of the primary solution, allowing the secondary or piggyback solution to flow when connected. Because manufacturers' designs vary, the nurse should check the directions carefully for the systems used in the agency. The nurse is responsible for calculating and manually adjusting the flow rate of the IV intermittent infusion or regulating the infusion with an infusion pump or controller.

Equipment

- Medication prepared in labeled small-volume bag or bottle
- Short secondary infusion tubing (microdrip or macrodrip)

Administering a Piggyback Intermittent Intravenous Infusion of Medication (continued)

- IV pump, if appropriate
- Needleless connector, stopcock, or sterile needle (21- to 23-gauge)
- Antimicrobial swab
- Tape (optional)
- Metal or plastic hook
- IV pole
- Date label for tubing
- Medication Administration Record (MAR) or Computer-generated MAR (CMAR)

ASSESSMENT

Assess the patient for any allergies. Check expiration date before administering medication. Assess the appropriateness of the drug for the patient. Assess the compatibility of the ordered medication, diluent, and the infusing IV fluid. Review assessment and laboratory data that may influence drug administration. Verify patient name, dose, route, and time of administration. Assess the patient's knowledge of the medication. If the patient has a knowledge deficit about the medication, this may be the appropriate time to begin education about the medication. If the medication may affect the patient's vital signs, assess them before administration. Assess the IV insertion site, noting any swelling, coolness, leakage of fluid at site, redness, or pain.

NURSING DIAGNOSIS

Determine related factors for the nursing diagnoses based on the patient's current status. Appropriate nursing diagnoses include:

- Acute Pain
- Risk for Allergy Response
- Risk for Injury
- Risk for Infection
- Deficient Knowledge

OUTCOME IDENTIFICATION AND PLANNING

The expected outcome to achieve is that the medication is delivered via the parenteral route using sterile technique. Other outcomes that may be appropriate include the following: medication is delivered to the patient in a safe manner and at the appropriate infusion rate; patient experiences no allergy response; patient remains infection free; and the patient understands and complies with the medication regimen.

IMPLEMENTATION

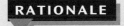
ACTION	RATIONALE

1. Gather equipment. Check each medication order against the original physician's order according to agency policy. Clarify any inconsistencies. Check the patient's chart for allergies.

This comparison helps to identify errors that may have occurred when orders were transcribed. The physician's order is the legal record of medication orders for each agency.

2. Know the actions, special nursing considerations, safe dose ranges, purpose of administration, and adverse effects of the medications to be administered. Consider the appropriateness of the medication for this patient.

This knowledge aids the nurse in evaluating the therapeutic effect of the medication in relation to the patient's disorder and can also be used to educate the patient about the medication.

3. Perform hand hygiene.

Hand hygiene prevents the spread of microorganisms.

(continued)

ACTION

RATIONALE

4. Move the medication cart to the outside of the patient's room or prepare for administration in the medication area.

Organization facilitates error-free administration and saves time.

5. Unlock the medication cart or drawer. Enter pass code and scan employee identification, if required.

Locking of the cart or drawer safeguards each patient's medication supply. Hospital accrediting organizations require medication carts to be locked when not in use. Entering pass code and scanning ID allows only authorized users into the system and identifies user for documentation by the computer.

6. **Prepare medications for one patient at a time.**

This prevents errors in medication administration.

7. Read the MAR and select the proper medication from the patient's medication drawer or unit stock.

This is the first check of the label.

8. Compare the label with the MAR. Check expiration dates. Confirm the prescribed or appropriate infusion rate. Calculate the drip rate if using gravity system. Scan the bar code on the package, if required.

This is the second check of the label. Verify calculations with another nurse to ensure safety, if necessary. Infusing medication at appropriate rate prevents injury.

9. **When all medications for one patient have been prepared, recheck the label with the MAR before taking them to the patient.**

This is a *third* check to ensure accuracy and to prevent errors.

10. Lock the medication cart before leaving it.

Locking the cart or drawer safeguards the patient's medication supply. Hospital accrediting organizations require medication carts to be locked when not in use.

11. Transport medications to the patient's bedside carefully, and keep the medications in sight at all times.

Careful handling and close observation prevent accidental or deliberate disarrangement of medications.

12. **Ensure that the patient receives the medications at the correct time.**

Check agency policy, which may allow for administration within a period of 30 minutes before or 30 minutes after designated time.

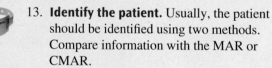 13. **Identify the patient.** Usually, the patient should be identified using two methods. Compare information with the MAR or CMAR.

Identifying the patient ensures the right patient receives the medications and helps prevent errors.

a. Check the name and identification number on the patient's identification band.

This is the most reliable method. Replace the identification band if it is missing or inaccurate in any way.

b. Ask the patient to state his or her name.

This requires a response from the patient, but illness and strange surroundings often cause patients to be confused.

c. If the patient cannot identify him or herself, verify the patient's identification with a staff member who knows the patient for the second source.

This is another way to double-check identity. Do not use the name on the door or over the bed, because these may be inaccurate.

14. Close the door to the room or pull the bedside curtain.

This provides patient privacy.

 15. Perform hand hygiene.

This prevents transmission of microorganisms.

Administering a Piggyback Intermittent Intravenous Infusion of Medication *(continued)*

ACTION	RATIONALE
16. Complete necessary assessments before administering medications. Check allergy bracelet or ask patient about allergies. Explain the purpose and action of the medication to the patient.	Assessment is a prerequisite to administration of medications. Explanation provides rationale, increases knowledge, and reduces anxiety.
17. Scan the patient's bar code on the identification band, if required.	Scanning provides an additional check to ensure that the medication is given to the right patient.
18. Assess the IV site for the presence of inflammation or infiltration.	IV medication must be given directly into a vein for safe administration.
19. Close the clamp on the short secondary infusion tubing. Using aseptic technique, remove the cap on the tubing spike and the cap on the port of the medication container, taking care to not contaminate either end.	Closing the clamp prevents fluid from entering system until the nurse is ready. Maintaining sterility of tubing and medication port prevents contamination.
20. Attach infusion tubing to the medication container by inserting the tubing spike into the port with a firm push and twisting motion, taking care to not contaminate either end.	Maintaining sterility of tubing and medication port prevents contamination.
21. **Hang piggyback container on IV pole, positioning it higher than primary IV according to manufacturer's recommendations (Figure 1).** Use metal or plastic hook to lower primary IV fluid container. (See the accompanying Skill Variation for information on administering an intermittent IV medication using a tandem piggyback set-up)	Position of containers influences the flow of IV fluid into primary setup.
22. Place label on tubing with appropriate date.	Tubing for piggyback setup may be used for 48 to 72 hours, depending on agency policy. Label allows for tracking of the next date to change.
23. Squeeze drip chamber and release. Fill to the line or about half full. Open clamp and prime tubing. Close clamp. Place needleless connector or needle on the end of the tubing, using sterile technique, if required.	This removes air from tubing and preserves sterility of setup.
24. Use an antimicrobial swab to clean the access port or stopcock above the roller clamp on the primary IV infusion tubing (Figure 2).	This deters entry of microorganisms when piggyback setup is connected to port.
25. Connect piggyback setup to the access port or stopcock (Figure 3). If using, turn the stopcock to the open position.	Needleless systems and stopcock setup eliminate the need for a needle and are recommended by the Centers for Disease Control and Prevention.
26. Use strip of tape to secure secondary tubing to primary infusion tubing, if a needle is used to connect.	Tape stabilizes needle in infusion port and prevents it from slipping out. Backflow valve in primary line secondary port stops flow of primary infusion while piggyback solution is infusing. Once completed, backflow valves opens and flow of primary solution resumes.
27. Open clamp on the secondary tubing. Use the roller clamp on the primary infusion tubing to regulate flow at prescribed delivery rate (Figure 4) or set rate for secondary infusion on infusion pump (Figure 5). Monitor medication infusion at periodic intervals.	Backflow valve in primary line secondary port stops flow of primary infusion while piggyback solution is infusing. Once completed, backflow valves opens and flow of primary solution resumes. It is important to verify the safe administration rate for each drug to prevent effects.

(continued)

Administering a Piggyback Intermittent Intravenous Infusion of Medication (continued)

ACTION

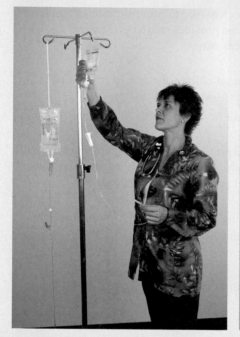

Figure 1. Positioning piggyback container on IV pole.

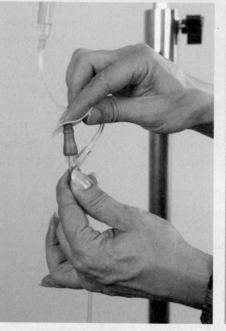

Figure 2. Cleaning access port.

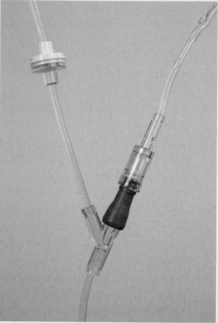

Figure 3. Connecting piggyback setup to access port.

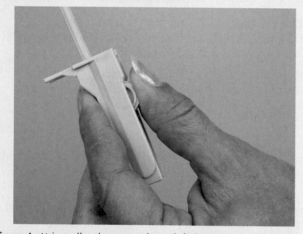

Figure 4. Using roller clamp on primary infusion tubing to regulate flow.

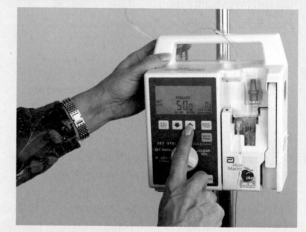

Figure 5. Adjusting pump rate.

28. Clamp tubing on piggyback set when solution is infused. Follow agency policy regarding disposal of equipment.

29. Replace primary IV fluid container to original height. **Readjust flow rate of primary IV or check primary infusion rate on infusion pump.**

RATIONALE

Most facilities allow the reuse of tubing for 48 to 72 hours. This reduces risk for contaminating primary IV setup.

Piggyback medication administration may interrupt normal flow rate of primary IV. Rate readjustment may be necessary. Many infusion pumps automatically restart primary infusion at previous rate after secondary infusion is completed.

ACTION	RATIONALE
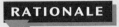 30. Perform hand hygiene.	Hand hygiene deters spread of microorganisms.
31. Evaluate patient's response to medication within appropriate time frame. Monitor IV site at periodic intervals.	Evaluate effectiveness of drug and provides early detection of adverse effect. Adverse reaction to medication given by the parenteral route is a possibility. Visualization of the site also allows for assessment of any untoward effects.

EVALUATION

The expected outcomes are met when the medication is delivered via the parenteral route using sterile technique; the medication is delivered to the patient in a safe manner and at the appropriate infusion rate; patient experiences no allergy response; patient remains infection free; and the patient understands and complies with the medication regimen.

DOCUMENTATION

Guidelines

Document the administration of the medication immediately after administration, including date, time, dose, route of administration, site of administration, and rate of administration on the MAR or record using the required format. If using a bar-code system, medication administration is automatically recorded when scanned. PRN medications require documentation of the reason for administration. Prompt recording avoids the possibility of accidentally repeating the administration of the drug. If the drug was refused or omitted, record this in the appropriate area on the medication record and notify the physician. This verifies the reason medication was omitted and ensures that the physician is aware of the patient's condition. Document the volume of fluid administered on the intake and output record, if necessary.

Unexpected Situations and Associated Interventions

- *Upon assessing the IV site before administering medication, the nurse notes that the IV has infiltrated:* Stop IV fluid and remove the IV from the extremity. Restart the IV in a different location. Continue to monitor the new IV site as medication is administered.
- *While administering medication, the nurse notes a cloudy, white substance forming in the IV tubing:* Stop the IV from flowing and stop administering the medication to prevent precipitate from entering the patient's circulation. Clamp the IV at the site nearest to the patient. Replace tubing on primary and secondary infusions. Check the literature regarding incompatibilities of medications before administering. Medication infusion may require second IV site or flushing of tubing before and after administration, using tandem system.
- *While nurse is administering medication, the patient begins to complain of pain at the IV site:* Stop the medication. Assess the IV site for any signs of infiltration or phlebitis. You may want to flush the IV with normal saline to check for patency. If the IV site appears within normal limits, resume medication administration at a slower rate.

Special Considerations

General Considerations

- An alternate way to prime the secondary tubing, particularly if administration set is in place from previous infusion, is to "backfill" the secondary tubing. Attach the medication bag to the secondary infusion tubing. Lower the medication bag below the main IV solution container and open the clamp on the secondary infusion tubing. This allows the primary IV solution to flow up the secondary tubing to the drip chamber, "backfilling" the tubing. Allow the solution to enter the drip chamber until the drip chamber is half full.

(continued)

Administering a Piggyback Intermittent Intravenous Infusion of Medication *(continued)*

Close the clamp on the secondary tubing and hang the medication container on the IV pole. Proceed with administration by lowering the primary IV container, as described above. This "backfill" method keeps the infusion system intact, preventing introduction of microorganisms and prevents loss of medication when the tubing is primed.

- Ongoing assessment is an important part of nursing care to evaluate patient response to administered medications and early detection of adverse effects. If an adverse effect is suspected, withhold further medication doses and notify the patient's primary healthcare provider. Additional intervention is based on type of reaction and patient assessment.

Infant and Child Considerations

- Small infants and children with fluid restrictions may not tolerate the added IV fluid needed for administration with piggyback or volume-control systems. For these children, consider using the mini-infusion pump.

SKILL VARIATION   Tandem Piggyback Setup

A tandem delivery setup allows for simultaneous infusion of the primary and secondary IV solutions. Both solution containers are hung at the same height. The tubing for the secondary infusion is attached to an access port below the roller clamp on the primary tubing. There is no back-check valve at the secondary port on the primary line. This type of setup is used infrequently because the solution from the primary IV line will back up into the tandem line if this intermittent infusion is not clamped immediately after it is infused.

- Check medication order against the original physician's order according to agency policy. Clarify any inconsistencies. Check the patient's chart for allergies. Verify the compatibility of the medication and IV fluid.
- Know the actions, special nursing considerations, safe dose ranges, purpose of administration, and adverse effects of the medications to be administered. Consider the appropriateness of the medication for this patient.
- Perform hand hygiene.
- Move the medication cart to the outside of the patient's room or prepare for administration in the medication area.
- Unlock the medication cart or drawer. Enter pass code and scan employee identification, if required.
- Read the MAR and select the proper medication from the patient's medication drawer or unit stock.
- Compare the label with the MAR. Check expiration dates. Confirm the prescribed or appropriate infusion rate. Calculate the drip rate if using gravity system. Scan the bar code on the package, if required.
- Recheck the label with the MAR before taking it to the patient.
- Lock the medication cart before leaving it.
- Transport medications and equipment to the patient's bedside carefully, and keep the medications in sight at all times.
- Perform hand hygiene.
- Identify the patient. Usually, the patient should be identified using two methods.
- Close the door to the room or pull the bedside curtain.
- Complete necessary assessments before administering medications. Check allergy bracelet or ask patient about allergies. Explain the purpose and action of the medication to the patient.

- Scan the patient's bar code on the identification band, if required.
- Assess the IV site for the presence of inflammation or infiltration.
- Close the clamp on the secondary infusion tubing. Using aseptic technique, remove the cap on the tubing spike and the cap on the port of the medication container, taking care to not contaminate either end.
- Attach infusion tubing to the medication container by inserting the tubing spike into the port with a firm push and twisting motion, taking care to not contaminate either end.
- Hang secondary container on IV pole, positioning it at the same height as the primary IV.
- Place label on tubing with appropriate date and attach needle or needleless device to end of tubing according to manufacturer's directions.
- Squeeze drip chamber and release. Fill to the line or about half full. Open clamp and prime tubing. Close clamp. Place needleless connector or needle on the end of the tubing, using sterile technique, if required.
- Use antimicrobial swab to clean the access port or stopcock below the roller clamp on the primary IV infusion tubing, usually the port closest to the IV insertion site.
- Connect secondary setup to the access port or stopcock. If using, turn the stopcock to the open position.
- Use strip of tape to secure secondary tubing to primary infusion tubing if a needle is used to connect.
- Use the roller clamp on the secondary infusion tubing to regulate flow at prescribed delivery rate. Monitor medication infusion at periodic intervals.
- Clamp tubing on secondary set when solution is infused. Remove secondary tubing from access port and replace connector or needle with a new capped one, if reusing. Follow agency policy regarding disposal of equipment.
- Check primary infusion rate.
- Perform hand hygiene.
- Evaluate patient's response to medication within appropriate time frame. Monitor IV site at periodic intervals.

Administering an Intermittent Intravenous Infusion of Medication via a Mini-Infusion Pump

With intermittent IV infusion, the drug is mixed with a small amount of the IV solution, such as 50 to 100 mL, and administered over a short period at the prescribed interval (eg, every 4 hours). Medication administration using an IV infusion pump requires the nurse to program the infusion rate into the pump. "Smart (computerized) pumps" are beginning to be used by many facilities for IV infusions, including intermittent infusions. "Smart pumps" also requiring programming of infusion rates by the nurse, but, in addition, are able to identify dosing limits and practice guidelines to aid in safe administration. Needleless devices (recommended by the Centers for Disease Control and Prevention and the Occupational Safety and Health Administration) prevent needlesticks and provide access to the primary venous line. Either blunt-ended cannulas or recessed connection ports may be used to connect intermittent IV infusions.

The mini-infusion pump (syringe pump) for intermittent infusion is battery or electrical operated and allows medication mixed in a syringe to be connected to the primary line and delivered by mechanical pressure applied to the syringe plunger (Figure 1).

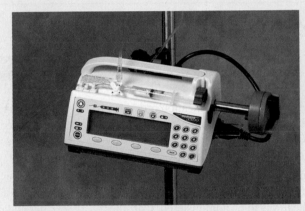

Figure 1. Syringe infusion pump.

Equipment

- Medication prepared in labeled syringe
- Mini-infusion pump and tubing
- Needleless connector, stopcock, or sterile needle (21- to 23-gauge)
- Antimicrobial swab
- Tape (optional)
- Date label for tubing
- Medication Administration Record (MAR) or Computer-generated MAR (CMAR)

ASSESSMENT

Assess the patient for any allergies. Check expiration date before administering medication. Assess the appropriateness of the drug for the patient. Assess the compatibility of the ordered medication, diluent, and the infusing IV fluid. Review assessment and laboratory data that may influence drug administration. Verify patient name, dose, route, and time of administration. Assess the patient's knowledge of the medication. If the patient has a knowledge deficit about the medication, this may be the appropriate time to begin education about the medication. If the medication may affect the patient's vital signs, assess them before administration. Assess the IV insertion site, noting any swelling, coolness, leakage of fluid at site, redness, or pain.

(continued)

NURSING DIAGNOSIS

Determine related factors for the nursing diagnoses based on the patient's current status. Appropriate nursing diagnoses include:

- Acute Pain
- Risk for Allergy Response
- Risk for Injury
- Risk for Infection
- Deficient Knowledge

OUTCOME IDENTIFICATION AND PLANNING

The expected outcome is that the medication is delivered via the parenteral route using sterile technique. Other outcomes that may be appropriate include the following: medication is delivered to the patient in a safe manner and at the appropriate infusion rate; patient experiences no allergy response; patient remains infection free; and the patient understands and complies with the medication regimen.

IMPLEMENTATION

ACTION

RATIONALE

1. Gather equipment. Check each medication order against the original physician's order according to agency policy. Clarify any inconsistencies. Check the patient's chart for allergies.

This comparison helps to identify errors that may have occurred when orders were transcribed. The physician's order is the legal record of medication orders for each agency.

2. Know the actions, special nursing considerations, safe dose ranges, purpose of administration, and adverse effects of the medications to be administered. Consider the appropriateness of the medication for this patient.

This knowledge aids the nurse in evaluating the therapeutic effect of the medication in relation to the patient's disorder and can also be used to educate the patient about the medication.

3. Perform hand hygiene.

Hand hygiene prevents the spread of microorganisms.

4. Move the medication cart to the outside of the patient's room or prepare for administration in the medication area.

Organization facilitates error-free administration and saves time.

5. Unlock the medication cart or drawer. Enter pass code and scan employee identification, if required.

Locking of the cart or drawer safeguards each patient's medication supply. Hospital accrediting organizations require medication carts to be locked when not in use. Entering pass code and scanning ID allows only authorized users into the system and identifies user for documentation by the computer.

6. **Prepare medications for one patient at a time.**

This prevents errors in medication administration.

7. Read the MAR and select the proper medication from the patient's medication drawer or unit stock.

This is the first check of the label.

8. Compare the label with the MAR. Check expiration dates. Confirm the prescribed or appropriate infusion rate. Calculate the drip rate if using gravity system. Scan the bar code on the package, if required.

This is the second check of the label. Verify calculations with another nurse to ensure safety, if necessary. Infusing medication at appropriate rate prevents injury.

Administering an Intermittent Intravenous Infusion of Medication via a Mini-Infusion Pump *(continued)*

ACTION	RATIONALE
9. **When all medications for one patient have been prepared, recheck the label with the MAR before taking them to the patient.**	This is the *third* check to ensure accuracy and to prevent errors.
10. Lock the medication cart before leaving it.	Locking the cart or drawer safeguards the patient's medication supply. Hospital accrediting organizations require medication carts to be locked when not in use.
11. Transport medications to the patient's bedside carefully, and keep the medications in sight at all times.	Careful handling and close observation prevent accidental or deliberate disarrangement of medications.
12. **Ensure that the patient receives the medications at the correct time.**	Check agency policy, which may allow for administration within a period of 30 minutes before or 30 minutes after designated time.
13. **Identify the patient.** Usually, the patient should be identified using two methods. Compare information with the MAR or CMAR.	Identifying the patient ensures the right patient receives the medications and helps prevent errors.
a. Check the name and identification number on the patient's identification band.	This is the most reliable method. Replace the identification band if it is missing or inaccurate in any way.
b. Ask the patient to state his or her name.	This requires a response from the patient, but illness and strange surroundings often cause patients to be confused.
c. If the patient cannot identify him or herself, verify the patient's identification with a staff member who knows the patient for the second source.	This is another way to double-check identity. Do not use the name on the door or over the bed, because these may be inaccurate.
14. Close the door to the room or pull the bedside curtain.	Provides patient privacy.
15. Perform hand hygiene.	Prevents transmission of microorganisms.
16. Complete necessary assessments before administering medications. Check allergy bracelet or ask patient about allergies. Explain the purpose and action of the medication to the patient.	Assessment is a prerequisite to administration of medications. Explanation provides rationale, increases knowledge, and reduces anxiety.
17. Scan the patient's bar code on the identification band, if required.	Provides additional check to ensure that the medication is given to the right patient.
18. Assess the IV site for the presence of inflammation or infiltration.	IV medication must be given directly into a vein for safe administration.
19. Using aseptic technique, remove the cap on the tubing and the cap on the syringe, taking care to not contaminate either end.	Maintaining sterility of tubing and syringe prevents contamination.
20. Attach infusion tubing to the syringe, taking care to not contaminate either end.	Maintaining sterility of tubing and medication port prevents contamination.
21. Place label on tubing with appropriate date and attach needle or needleless device to end of tubing according to manufacturer's directions.	Tubing for piggyback setup may be used for 48 to 72 hours, depending on agency policy. Label allows for tracking of the next date to change.

(continued)

SKILL 12

Administering an Intermittent Intravenous Infusion of Medication via a Mini-Infusion Pump *(continued)*

ACTION	**RATIONALE**
22. Fill tubing with medication by applying gentle pressure to syringe plunger. Place needleless connector or needle on the end of the tubing, using sterile technique, if required.	This removes air from tubing and maintains sterility.
23. Insert syringe into mini-infusion pump according to manufacturer's directions.	Syringe must fit securely in pump apparatus for proper operation.
24. Use antimicrobial swab to clean the access port or stopcock below the roller clamp on the primary IV infusion tubing, usually the port closest to the IV insertion site.	This deters entry of microorganisms when piggyback setup is connected to port. Proper connection allows IV medication to flow into primary line.
25. Connect the secondary infusion to the primary infusion at the cleansed port.	Allows for delivery of medication.
26. Program pump to the appropriate rate and begin infusion. Set alarm if recommended by manufacturer.	Pump delivers medication at controlled rate. Alarm is recommended for use with IV lock apparatus.
27. Clamp tubing on secondary set when solution is infused. Remove secondary tubing from access port and replace connector or needle with a new, capped one, if reusing. Follow agency policy regarding disposal of equipment.	Many facilities allow reuse of tubing for 48 to 72 hours. Replacing connector or needle with a new, capped one maintains sterility of system.
28. Check rate of primary infusion.	Administration of secondary infusion may interfere with primary infusion rate.
29. Perform hand hygiene.	Hand hygiene deters spread of microorganisms.
30. Evaluate patient's response to medication within appropriate time frame. Monitor IV site at periodic intervals.	Evaluate effectiveness of drug and provides early detection of adverse effect. Adverse reaction to medication given by the parenteral route is a possibility. Visualization of the site also allows for assessment of any untoward effects.

EVALUATION

The expected outcomes are met when the medication is delivered via the parenteral route using sterile technique; the medication is delivered to the patient in a safe manner and at the appropriate infusion rate; patient experiences no allergy response; patient remains infection free; and the patient understands and complies with the medication regimen.

DOCUMENTATION

Guidelines

Document the administration of the medication immediately after administration, including date, time, dose, route of administration, site of administration, and rate of administration on the MAR or record using the required format. If using a bar-code system, medication administration is automatically recorded when scanned. PRN medications require documentation of the reason for administration. Prompt recording avoids the possibility of accidentally repeating the administration of the drug. If the drug was refused or omitted, record this in the appropriate area on the medication record and notify the physician. This verifies the reason medication was omitted and ensures that the physician is aware of the patient's condition. Document the volume of fluid administered on the intake and output record, if necessary.

Administering an Intermittent Intravenous Infusion of Medication via a Mini-Infusion Pump *(continued)*

Special Considerations

General Considerations

- Ongoing assessment is an important part of nursing care to evaluate patient response to administered medications and early detection of adverse effects. If an adverse effect is suspected, withhold further medication doses and notify the patient's primary healthcare provider. Additional intervention is based on type of reaction and patient assessment.

Administering an Intermittent Intravenous Infusion of Medication via a Volume-Control Administration Set

With intermittent IV infusion, the drug is mixed with a small amount of the IV solution, such as 50 to 100 mL, and administered over a short period at the prescribed interval (eg, every 4 hours). Administration is achieved by gravity infusion, which requires the nurse to calculate the infusion rate in drops per minute. This skill discusses using a volume-control administration set for intermittent IV infusion. The medication is diluted with a small amount of solution and administered through the patient's IV line. This type of equipment is commonly used for infusing solutions into children, critically ill, and older patients when the volume of fluid infused is a concern. Needleless devices (recommended by the Centers for Disease Control and Prevention and the Occupational Safety and Health Administration) prevent needlesticks and provide access to the primary venous line. Either a blunt-ended cannula or a recessed connection port may be used to connect intermittent IV infusions.

Equipment

- Prescribed medication
- Syringe with a 19- to 21-gauge needle, blunt needle or needleless device (follow agency policy)
- Volume-control set (Volutrol®, Buretrol®, Burette®)
- Needleless connector, stopcock, or sterile needle (21- to 23-gauge)
- Antimicrobial swab
- Tape (optional)
- Date label for tubing
- Medication label
- Medication Administration Record (MAR) or Computer-generated MAR (CMAR)

ASSESSMENT

Assess the patient for any allergies. Check expiration date before administering medication. Assess the appropriateness of the drug for the patient. Assess the compatibility of the ordered medication, diluent, and the infusing IV fluid. Review assessment and laboratory data that may influence drug administration. Assess the patient's knowledge of the medication. If the patient has a knowledge deficit about the medication, this may be the appropriate time to begin education about the medication. If the medication may affect the patient's vital signs, assess them before administration. Assess the IV insertion site, noting any swelling, coolness, leakage of fluid at site, redness, or pain.

NURSING DIAGNOSIS

Determine related factors for the nursing diagnoses based on the patient's current status. Appropriate nursing diagnoses include:

- Acute Pain
- Risk for Allergy Response
- Risk for Injury
- Risk for Infection
- Deficient Knowledge

(continued)

Administering an Intermittent Intravenous Infusion of Medication via a Volume-Control Administration Set *(continued)*

OUTCOME IDENTIFICATION AND PLANNING

The expected outcome to achieve when administering an intermittent IV infusion of medication via a volume control set is that the medication is delivered via the parenteral route using sterile technique. Other outcomes that may be appropriate include the following: medication is delivered to the patient in a safe manner and at the appropriate infusion rate; patient experiences no allergy response; patient remains infection free; and the patient understands and complies with the medication regimen.

IMPLEMENTATION

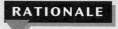

ACTION	RATIONALE
1. Gather equipment. Check medication order against the original physician's order according to agency policy. Clarify any inconsistencies. Check the patient's chart for allergies. Verify the compatibility of the medication and IV fluid.	This comparison helps to identify errors that may have occurred when orders were transcribed. The physician's order is the legal record of medication orders for each agency. Compatibility of medication and solution prevents complications.
2. Know the actions, special nursing considerations, safe dose ranges, purpose of administration, and adverse effects of the medications to be administered. Consider the appropriateness of the medication for this patient.	This knowledge aids the nurse in evaluating the therapeutic effect of the medication in relation to the patient's disorder and can also be used to educate the patient about the medication.
3. Perform hand hygiene.	Hand hygiene prevents the spread of microorganisms.
4. Move the medication cart to the outside of the patient's room or prepare for administration in the medication area.	Organization facilitates error-free administration and saves time.
5. Unlock the medication cart or drawer. Enter pass code and scan employee identification, if required.	Locking of the cart or drawer safeguards each patient's medication supply. Hospital accrediting organizations require medication carts to be locked when not in use. Entering pass code and scanning ID allows only authorized users into the system and identifies user for documentation by the computer.
6. **Prepare medication for one patient at a time.**	This prevents errors in medication administration.
7. Read the MAR and select the proper medication from the patient's medication drawer or unit stock.	This is the first check of the label.
8. Compare the label with the MAR. Check expiration dates and perform calculations, if necessary. Scan the bar code on the package, if required. Check the infusion rate.	This is the second check of the label. Verify calculations with another nurse to ensure safety, if necessary. Delivers the correct dose of medication as prescribed.
9. If necessary, withdraw medication from an ampule or vial as described in Skills 2 and 3. Attach needleless connector or needle to end of syringe, if necessary.	Allows for entry into the volume-control administration set chamber.
10. **Recheck the label with the MAR before taking it to the patient.**	This is a *third* check to ensure accuracy and to prevent errors.

SKILL
13

Administering an Intermittent Intravenous Infusion of Medication via a Volume-Control Administration Set *(continued)*

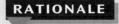

ACTION	**RATIONALE**
11. Prepare medication label including name of medication, dose, total volume, including diluent, and time of administration.	Allows for accurate identification of medication.
12. Lock the medication cart before leaving it.	Locking the cart or drawer safeguards the patient's medication supply. Hospital accrediting organizations require medication carts to be locked when not in use.
13. Transport medications and equipment to the patient's bedside carefully, and keep the medications in sight at all times.	Careful handling and close observation prevent accidental or deliberate disarrangement of medications. Having equipment available saves time and facilitates performance of the task.
14. Perform hand hygiene.	Hand hygiene deters the spread of microorganisms.
15. **Identify the patient.** Usually, the patient should be identified using two methods. Compare information with the MAR or CMAR.	Identifying the patient ensures the right patient receives the medications and helps prevent errors.
a. Check the name and identification number on the patient's identification band.	This is the most reliable method. Replace the identification band if it is missing or inaccurate in any way.
b. Ask the patient to state his or her name.	This requires a response from the patient, but illness and strange surroundings often cause patients to be confused.
c. If the patient cannot identify him or herself, verify the patient's identification with a staff member who knows the patient for the second source.	This is another way to double-check identity. Do not use the name on the door or over the bed, because these may be inaccurate.
16. Close the door to the room or pull the bedside curtain.	This provides patient privacy.
17. Complete necessary assessments before administering medications. Check allergy bracelet or ask patient about allergies. Explain the purpose and action of the medication to the patient.	Assessment is a prerequisite to administration of medications. Explanation provides rationale, increases knowledge, and reduces anxiety.
18. Scan the patient's bar code on the identification band, if required.	Provides additional check to ensure that the medication is given to the right patient.
19. **Assess IV site for presence of inflammation or infiltration.**	IV medication must be given directly into a vein for safe administration.
20. Fill the volume-control administration set (Figure 1) with the prescribed amount of IV fluid by opening the clamp between IV solution and the volume-control administration set. Follow manufacturer's instructions and fill with prescribed amount of IV solution (Figure 2). Close clamp.	This dilutes the medication in the minimal amount of solution. Reclamping prevents the continued addition of fluid to the volume to be mixed with medication.
21. Check to make sure the air vent on the volume-control administration set chamber is open.	Air vent allows fluid in the chamber to flow at a regular rate.
22. Use antimicrobial swab to clean access port on volume-control administration set chamber (Figure 3).	This deters entry of microorganisms when the syringe enters chamber.

(continued)

SKILL 13

Administering an Intermittent Intravenous Infusion of Medication via a Volume-Control Administration Set *(continued)*

ACTION

RATIONALE

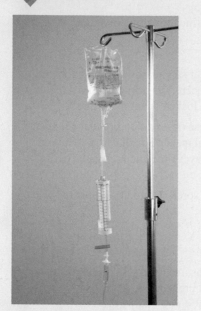

Figure 1. Volume-control administration set and IV solution for dilution of medication.

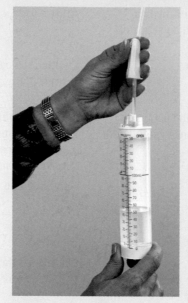

Figure 2. Opening clamp between IV solution and volume-control administration set to fill chamber with prescribed amount of solution.

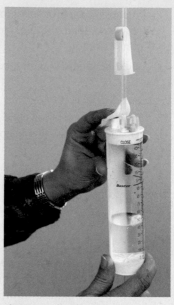

Figure 3. Cleaning access port.

23. Insert the needle or blunt needleless device into port while holding syringe steady (Figure 4). Inject medication into the chamber (Figure 5). Gently rotate the chamber.

This ensures that medication is evenly mixed with solution.

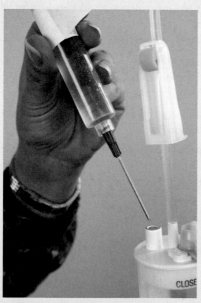

Figure 4. Inserting needleless device into port.

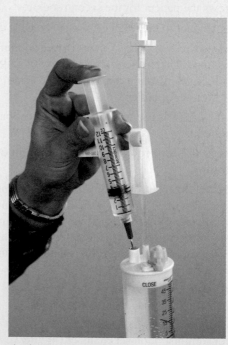

Figure 5. Injecting the medication into the volume-control device.

Administering an Intermittent Intravenous Infusion of Medication via a Volume-Control Administration Set *(continued)*

ACTION	**RATIONALE**
24. Attach the medication label to the volume-control device (Figure 6).	This identifies contents of the set and prevents medication error.
25. Use antimicrobial swab to clean the access port or stopcock below the roller clamp on the primary IV infusion tubing, usually the port closest to the IV insertion site.	This deters entry of microorganisms when piggyback setup is connected to port. Proper connection allows IV medication to flow into primary line.
26. Connect the secondary infusion to the primary infusion at the cleansed port.	This allows for delivery of medication.
27. Use the roller clamp on the volume-control administration set tubing to adjust the infusion to the prescribed rate (Figure 7).	Delivery over a 30- to 60-minute interval is a safe method of administering IV medication.

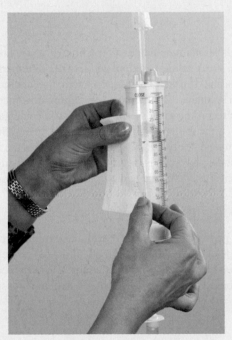

Figure 6. Applying medication label to volume-control device.

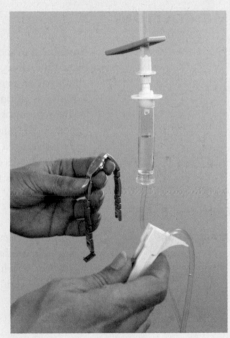

Figure 7. Using roller clamp on volume-control administration set to adjust medication infusion rate.

28. Do not recap the used needle. Engage the safety shield or needle guard, if present. Discard the needle and syringe in the appropriate receptacle.	Proper disposal of the needle prevents injury.
29. Clamp tubing on secondary set when solution is infused. Remove secondary tubing from access port and replace connector or needle with a new, capped one, if reusing. Follow agency policy regarding disposal of equipment.	Many facilities allow reuse of tubing for 48 to 72 hours. Replacing connector or needle with a new, capped one maintains sterility of system.
30. Check rate of primary infusion.	Administration of secondary infusion may interfere with primary infusion rate.
31. Perform hand hygiene.	Hand hygiene deters spread of microorganisms.

(continued)

Administering an Intermittent Intravenous Infusion of Medication via a Volume-Control Administration Set *(continued)*

ACTION

RATIONALE

32. Evaluate patient's response to medication within appropriate time frame. Monitor IV site at periodic intervals.

Evaluates effectiveness of drug and provides early detection of adverse effect. Adverse reaction to medication given by the parenteral route is a possibility. Visualization of the site also allows for assessment of any untoward effects.

EVALUATION

The expected outcomes are met when the medication is delivered via the parenteral route using sterile technique; the medication is delivered to the patient in a safe manner and at the appropriate infusion rate; patient experiences no allergy response; patient remains infection free; and the patient understands and complies with the medication regimen.

DOCUMENTATION

Guidelines

Document the administration of the medication immediately after administration, including date, time, dose, route of administration, site of administration, and rate of administration on the MAR or record using the required format. If using a bar-code system, medication administration is automatically recorded when scanned. PRN medications require documentation of the reason for administration. Prompt recording avoids the possibility of accidentally repeating the administration of the drug. If the drug was refused or omitted, record this in the appropriate area on the medication record and notify the physician. This verifies the reason medication was omitted and ensures that the physician is aware of the patient's condition. Document the volume of fluid administered on the intake and output record, if necessary.

Special Considerations

General Considerations

• Ongoing assessment is an important part of nursing care to evaluate patient response to administered medications and early detection of adverse effects. If an adverse effect is suspected, withhold further medication doses and notify the patient's primary healthcare provider. Additional intervention is based on type of reaction and patient assessment.